Comprehensive Summaries of Uppsala Dissertations
from the Faculty of Medicine   1065

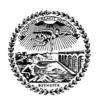

Needs Assessment in Occupational Therapy

Studies of Persons with Long-Term/Recurrent Pain

BY

MARIA MÜLLERSDORF

ACTA UNIVERSITATIS UPSALIENSIS
UPPSALA 2001

Dissertation for the Degree of Doctor of Philosophy (Faculty of Medicine) in Caring Sciences presented at Uppsala University in 2001

ABSTRACT

Müllersdorf, M. 2001. Needs Assessment in Occupational Therapy. Studies of Persons with Long-Term/Recurrent Pain. Acta Universitatis Upsaliensis. *Comprehensive Summaries of Uppsala Dissertations from the Faculty of Medicine* 1065. 88 pp. Uppsala. ISBN 91-554-5086-5.

The overall aim of this thesis is to describe (1) needs/problems among persons with self-perceived activity limitations and/or participation restrictions due to long-term/recurrent pain, and (2) treatment interventions in occupational therapy to meet demonstrated needs. A randomly selected sample (n=10,000) from the Swedish general population aged 18-58 years was the foundation of the study population including persons with and without pain. In addition, occupational therapists were included (n=109). Data collection was made by postal questionnaires. The results showed a prevalence of 26 % and an incidence rate of 0.07 for self-perceived activity limitations/participation restrictions due to long-term/recurrent pain. There were more women in the age group 40-58 years with short education among persons with pain. Pain in shoulders/lower back of searing/aching/gnawing character was the most frequently reported. A majority of the respondents reported affective/emotional effects of pain mainly of a depressive character and they had previously been on sick leave due to pain. Women reported higher frequencies of self-perceived activity limitations/participation restrictions due to pain, more difficulties with intermediate ADL, perceived higher job demands and had longer sick leave than men. Men perceived poorer social support than did women. Needs for occupational therapy were reported mainly as limitations in activity performance and temporal imbalance. High health care consumers reported higher frequencies of needs/problems than did low health care consumers. The main goals and interventions suggested by occupational therapists to meet the needs in pain management focused on increased knowledge of handling daily occupations with the purpose to reduce pain, maintain competence/improve performance of home maintenance, reduce the consequences of pain and increase knowledge about how to handle effects of pain.

Key words: Needs assessment, occupational therapy, long-term/recurrent pain, activity limitations/participation restrictions.

Maria Müllersdorf, Department of Public Health and Caring Sciences, Section of Caring Sciences, Uppsala University, Uppsala Science Park, SE 751 83 Uppsala, Sweden

ISSN 0282-7476
ISBN 91-554-5086-5

Printed in Sweden by Uppsala University, Tryck & Medier, Uppsala 2001

Need, like beauty,
is in the eye of the
beholder (M. Cooper)

ORIGINAL PUBLICATIONS

This thesis is based on the following papers that are referred to in the text by their Roman numerals.

I.   Müllersdorf, M., Söderback, I. (2000). Assessing health care needs: the actual state of self-perceived activity limitation and participation restrictions due to pain in a nationwide Swedish population. *International Journal of Rehabilitation Research,* **23**: 201-207.

II.   Müllersdorf, M., Söderback, I. (2000). The actual state of the effects, treatment and incidence of disabling pain in a gender perspective – a Swedish study. *Disability and Rehabilitation,* **22**: 840-854.

III.   Müllersdorf, M. (2000). Factors indicating need of rehabilitation – occupational therapy among persons with long-term and/or recurrent pain. *International Journal of Rehabilitation Research,* **23**: 281-294.

IV.   Müllersdorf, M., Söderback, I. (2001). Occupational therapists' assessments of adults with long-term pain, the Swedish experience. *Occupational Therapy International*. Accepted for publication.

V.   Müllersdorf, M. Needs/problems related to occupational therapy among adult Swedes with long-term pain. Manuscript.

Reprints were made with permission of the publishers.

ACTA UNIVERSITATIS UPSALIENSIS
Comprehensive Summaries of Uppsala Dissertations from the Faculty of Medicine 1065
Distributor: Uppsala University Library, Box 510, SE-751 20 Uppsala, Sweden

Maria Müllersdorf
Needs Assessment in Occupational Therapy.
Studies of Persons with Long-Term/ Recurrent Pain

Akademisk avhandling som för avläggande av medicine doktorsexamen i Omvårdnadsforskning vid Uppsala Universitet, kommer att offentligt försvaras i universitetshusets lärosal X, fredagen den 28 september 2001 kl. 9.00

ABSTRACT
Müllersdorf, M. 2001. Needs Assessment in Occupational Therapy. Studies of Persons with Long-Term/Recurrent Pain. Acta Universitatis Upsaliensis. *Comprehensive Summaries of Uppsala Dissertations from the Faculty of Medicine* 1065. 88 pp. Uppsala. ISBN 91-554-5086-5.

The overall aim of this thesis was to describe (1) needs for occupational therapy among persons with self-perceived activity limitations and/or participation restrictions due to long-term/recurrent pain, and (2) treatment interventions in occupational therapy to meet demonstrated needs. The Liss' model for assessing health care needs was used as a structural scheme. A randomly selected sample (n=10,000) from the Swedish general population aged 18-58 years was the foundation for the study population with and without pain. In addition, occupational therapists were included (n=109). Data collection was made by postal questionnaires. The results showed a prevalence of 26 % and an incidence rate of 0.07. Demographic characteristics of the sample were female gender, ages 40-58 years and fewer years of education than those without pain. Pain in shoulders/lower back of searing/aching/gnawing character was the most frequently reported. A majority of the respondents reported affective/emotional effects of pain mainly of depressive character and they had previously been on sick leave due to pain. Women reported higher frequencies of self-perceived activity limitations/ participation restrictions due to pain, more difficulties with intermediate ADL, perceived higher job demands and had longer sick leave than men. Men perceived poorer social support than did women. Needs for occupational therapy were reported mainly as a consequence of activity and temporal imbalance. High health care consumers reported higher frequencies of needs/problems than did low health care consumers. The main goals and interventions suggested by occupational therapists to meet the needs in pain management focused on increased knowledge of handling daily occupations with the purpose to reduce pain, maintain competence/improve performance of home maintenance, reduce consequences of pain and increase knowledge how to handle effects of pain.

Key words: Needs assessment, occupational therapy, long-term/recurrent pain, activity limitations/participation restrictions.

Maria Müllersdorf, Department of Public Health and Caring Sciences, Section of Caring Sciences, Uppsala University, Uppsala Science Park, SE 751 83 Uppsala, Sweden

CONTENTS

INTRODUCTION

When community financial resources are reduced and the need and demand for health services are increasing, needs assessment becomes a priority issue in health care for politicians, care providers, managers and employees (SOU, 1995). It becomes important to develop methods and guidelines to ensure that resources will be effectively used and for the "right" patients (SOS, 1999). To that end, criteria should be mapped that reflect characteristics of a group of persons/patients (Joe, 1991; Söderback, 1993; Wright & Whittington, 1992), that can be used to distinguish those who have the most benefit from specific health care interventions (e.g. occupational therapy) (SOS, 1999). At present there are no Swedish guidelines concerning for whom occupational therapy would be beneficial within the patient-category of working age with long-term/recurrent pain (SOU, 2000). Whether patients are referred to occupational therapy or not seems to depend on the referring part's knowledge about occupational therapy, current health care, rehabilitation routines, county-council policy and on the different perspectives within the health care disciplines (Andersson, 1997; Jensen et al, 2000; Söderback et al, 2000, Turner et al, 1998). When establishing health care priorities, needs assessments may be helpful (Polit & Hungler, 1995) to distinguish persons who may benefit from occupational therapy. This would probably be of advantage for the patient, for an optimal use of health care and for society (Fishbain et al, 1996; Linton & Hallden, 1998; SOS, 1999).

Needs as a concept

Although the concept of need seems intuitive, it is defined in several, partly contradictory ways and as Soriano (1995) puts it " ......*it is technical and sophisticated*". Liss (1990) describes three aspects of need: (1) need as a difference (a teleological need), "P doesn't have x"; (2) need as a state of tension, "P has a need" which means that P has a drive to get x; and (3) need as an object "x is a need of P's". Need can also be classified by associated goals. Thus, Benn and Peters (1964) list (1) biological needs – for survival; (2) basic needs – for a person to reach a decent state of living, and (3) functional needs – what is needed to do a particular job. Bunston et al

1

(1994) distinguish between expressed and unexpressed need, while Simeone, Frank and Aryan (1993) distinguish between met and unmet demand with a focus on received treatment. Matthew (1971) stated that need for medical care exists when a person has an illness or disability for which an effective and acceptable treatment was provided. In a literature review of needs assessments methods in health care, it was suggested that Benn and Peter's definition of basic and functional needs would probably be of use for the field of occupational therapy, as would Bunston's unresolved and unexpressed need: *"daily life tasks as a focus in occupational therapy seem often to be unresolved or unexpressed..."* (p.71) (Müllersdorf & Söderback, 1998). In sum, patients/clients may be aware of their needs. These needs are recognized, can be expressed and can be met or unmet. Professionals or others may observe patients' needs, both those recognized as those unrecognised by the patient. The unrecognised needs are those that patients are not aware of and that are therefore not expressed by them. Unrecognised and unexpressed needs are most often unmet (Figure 1).

Patients / clients	Recognized needs	Expressed needs	Met needs
Professionals or others			Unmet needs
Professionals or others	Unrecognised needs	Not expressed needs	Met needs
			Unmet needs

Figure 1: An overview of some ways to classify patient/client needs.

Needs assessment – methods in health care and rehabilitation

Needs assessments may be performed in various ways (Müllersdorf & Söderback, 1998) to describe individual as well as community needs (Liss, 1990, Wright et al, 1998). According to Bunston et al (1994), assessing patients' need is essential for three reasons;

- *"The use of health services is related to the specific needs of specific populations during specific periods,*
- *meeting psychosocial needs improves medical outcomes, and*

- *patient's and professional caregiver's reports of patients' needs are often in-congruent and diminish the use of services."* (p. 227)

As well as stating that needs assessment may be a priority issue and that there are no guidelines, Royce and Drude (1982) add *"almost anything can pass for a needs as-sessment"* (p. 97). However, this does not mean that there is a total lack of guidelines for assessment of needs.

Information about specific needs should be collected from individual clients/pa-tients or key informants with special knowledge of the area (Balacki, 1988; Liss, 1990; Percy-Smith, 1996; Soriano, 1995). Some authors claim that disabled persons often are the best source of information about their own lives (Bunston et al, 1994; Burnett & Yerxa, 1980). Manderbacka (1998) concludes: *"... to the extent that health is measured as an individual experience and not only as absence or presence of a medically defined pathology, the individual is probably the best (if not the only) per-son to judge it."* (p. 9) On the other hand, it has been pointed out that patients may have trouble to express their concerns (Bunston & Mings, 1995). Jensen et al (2000) found that experts (physicians, physiotherapists and social insurance officers) based their judgements only on the patients' age and not on health-related aspects when assessing need and potential for rehabilitation. The most consistent predictor of health and work status was the patients' own belief in effective treatments and her ability to learn to cope with the situation. Thus, needs may be valued in different ways by the patient and the caregiver, despite having access to the same information. This indicates the value of having several sources and methods when collecting and interpreting data (Bunston & Mings, 1995; Kresten et al, 2000; SOU, 1995; Turner et al, 1998). When individual clients/patients are the main sources, interviews and ques-tionnaires are suggested for data collection (Soriano, 1995).

Assessment of need is never free of values, and may be performed in various ways. Thus, there is no "golden standard", why the main point is to find the most ap-propriate method for the particular circumstances at hand (Wilkin, 1993). Needs as-sessments have been recommended as a starting point for any treatment intervention in health care (Lawton, 1999).

A model for needs assessment in health care

Liss (1990) recommends a model for assessing health care needs applicable both to individuals and populations. This model states that there is a health care need when a difference exists between the actual state of health and the goal of health, and health care treatments are necessary to reduce or eliminate the difference. A need may be satisfied when the actual state is changed towards the goals. In this model, health is related to the individuals ability to reach vital goals. The model includes three steps: (1) the actual state, (2) the goal of health care need and (3) the object of health care need.

The first step *"establish the actual state"* gives information about health status and indicates the magnitude of the problem. Information about the actual state is based on empirical observations. The next step *"settle the goal of health care need"* refers either to the patients' or the health care providers' goal(s) for health care. That is, the goal refers to what should be achieved (e.g. reduce pain, be able to perform activities). The goal(s) are chosen by the patients and/or the caregivers. Information about the difference between the actual state and the goal of health is necessary for identification of health care needs. However, goals may be expressed in very general terms. One way to determine goals is ask the respondents to identify their needs and thereby implicitly identify adequate goals. The final step, *"determine the object of need"* refers to the treatments that would be necessary to meet health-related needs, or in other words, to reach the goals. An assessment of possible treatments also requires information about expected effects. When assessing the health status of a population, Liss suggests survey studies of a representative sample using questionnaires or interviews for data collection.

The Liss' model for assessing health care needs will be used to structure the present thesis.

Assessing needs by questionnaires

Questionnaires are frequently recommended for data collection when assessing health care needs (e.g. Liss, 1990; Wilkin 1993; Wright et al, 1998) and are reported to provide reliable data for the determination of rehabilitation needs (Bruhn & Trevino, 1979; Burnett & Yerxa, 1980). Needs assessment instruments for different areas of health care have been described in the literature (e.g. Bruhn & Trevino, 1979; Dragone 1990; Kent et al, 2000; Kresten et al, 2000; Wilkin, 1993) and the construction of instruments varies. Mainly two types of questions are represented in the instruments. The first type asks the respondents about their needs in a straight-forward way, for example what health care services the patient desires (Warms, 1987), their need for assistance in activities of daily living (Reviere et al, 1994), or their need to talk with somebody about their problems (Bruhn & Trevino, 1979). This type of questions would probably detect needs that are recognized and expressed by the respondents. The second type of questions concerns problems and are expressed as questions or statements, e.g. The Cancer Needs Survey in which questions about psychological, social and economic problems are included (Houldin & Wasserbauer, 1996). Other examples are a questionnaire for parents about their children's health problems (Rustia et al, 1984), the Primary Health Care Needs Assessment with statements about young people's problems (Dragone, 1990), and The Occupational Therapy Needs Assessment with questions about cancer patients' problems in daily activities (Söderback & Hammersly-Paulsson, 1997; Söderback et al, 2000). Well-known and standardized instruments like the Sickness Impact Profile has also been used for need assessment (Wilkin, 1993). The second type of questions about patient problems would probably yield information about needs not recognized or expressed as such by the respondents.

Criteria as a selection tool

Criteria reflecting characteristics that are specific for a group of persons/patients, who have reported needs/problems in greater frequencies than others, might be used as a tool to select patients for specific treatments (Joe, 1991; Söderback, 1993; Wright & Whittington, 1992). This is in line with the database MedLine statement: *"Criteria and standards used for the determination of the appropriateness of the inclusion of patients with specific conditions in proposed treatment plans..."* (Med-Line, 2000).

Examples of criteria for patient selection are psycho-social characteristics used for inclusion in cardiac procedures as an indicator of need for special interventions (Giacomini et al, 2001), and the use of the body mass index and cardiovascular disease as selection criteria for weight-loss treatment (Kiernan & Winkleby, 2000). Specific characteristics of the target population may be assessed by survey methods (Brink & Wood, 1989). Such characteristics specific for the group of persons/patients of interest could be used as independent variables in statistical regression analyses to predict outcome variables (Tabachnick & Fidell, 1996). If the specific characteristics of a target population are valid as selection criteria for treatment must be evaluated in controlled clinical studies (Kazdin, 1998).

Occupational therapy

A central assumption in occupational therapy is a focus on the individual's right to a meaningful and productive life, despite chronic disease (Mosey, 1974; 1996). The overall aim of occupational therapy is to prevent disability (Jacobs, 1999; Stein & Rose, 2000) and enable function and well-being in everyday occupations (Hopkins & Smith, 1993; Jacobs, 1999; Reed & Sanderson, 1999; Stein & Rose, 2000) by the therapeutic use of purposeful activities (Reed & Sanderson 1999; Stein & Rose 2000). Reed and Sanderson (1999) define the unique aspects of occupational therapy as; *"Application of the knowledge of occupation to assist persons to develop, learn, and maintain occupational performance... and Application of methods (called also techniques or approaches) of adapting and changing a person's occupational behaviour to meet the demands of the human and nonhuman environments (environmental press) or adapting and changing the environment to a person's occupational needs."* (1999, p 57).

Occupational therapy is described in terms of a health-oriented, rather than a medical discipline, as the focus is on the effects of a disease or an injury on everyday living (Christiansen & Baum, 1997; Törnquist, 1995). In rehabilitation, in which occupational therapy is represented, the goal is to prevent or reduce effects of disability (i.e. the activity perspective). This contrast with medicine, the goal of which is to restore structures or functions (i.e. the impairment perspective) (Schut & Stam,

1994). The occupational therapist, as a member of the rehabilitation team, contributes with her/his professional specific knowledge, skills and working methods (Bellner, 1997) grounded in activity as a goal but also as a tool (Mosey 1996; Reed & Sanderson 1999; Tjornov, 1987; Törnquist, 1995).

Historically, occupational therapy in Sweden was represented in psychiatric health care and tuberculosis sanatoria already in the 19th century, but the entrance in other somatic health care with more regularity occurred in the middle of the 20th century (Björklund, 2000; Lindström, 1990; Lund & Andersson-Nordberg 1998). Occupational therapy is thus a young profession and its development can be illustrated in terms of the following phases. One period was reductionistic (1970-1977) which developed towards a humanistic/holistic period (1977-1983). The following decade was a phase of deepening in both reductionism and holism (Lund & Andersson-Nordberg, 1998). The present period seems to be influenced by the concepts of occupation/activity, meaning that the occupational therapist will approach the patient with a focus on activity limitation rather than with a diagnostic perspective (Björklund, 2000).

Occupation, activity and occupations in daily life
The concepts of occupation and activity are often used synonymously and various definitions can be found in the literature. Several authors emphasise that the concept of occupation should be used rather than activity, as the former is more expressive and encompassing (Christiansen & Baum, 1997; Darnell & Heater, 1994; Nelson 1997). Occupation has been defined by Clark et al (1998) as daily activities that can be named in the lexicon of a culture. Another definition of occupation is described as the relationship between occupational performance and occupational form. Occupational performance is the doing and occupational form is the context that is external to the person, i.e. materials, environment, other persons, temporal dimensions and socio-cultural reality together constituting the act with purpose and meaning (Nelson, 1997). The concept of occupation may include several activities and therefore seems to be a more comprehensive concept than activity (Hinojosa & Kramer, 1997). In Sweden there is no consensus about how the terms "activity" and "occupation"

should be used. Translation into other languages (e.g. Swedish) is difficult because it requires sorting out the differences between the concepts and no suitable words may be available why occupation and activity are often used interchangeably (Björklund, 2000).

Occupations in daily life, often described as activities in daily life (ADL), include the things humans do daily or with some regularity e.g. self-care, house-management, work and leisure (Törnquist, 1995). Several authors divide the concept in two parts – personal/self-care activities and instrumental activities (Christiansen & Baum, 1997; Trombly, 1995). Self-care activities are defined as: *"activities or tasks done routinely to maintain the clients health and well-being, considering the environment and social factors"* (Trombly, 1995, p. 352) (e.g. toileting, bathing, dressing, eating etc), while instrumental activities are *"more complex activities of tasks a person does to maintain independence in the home and community"* (Trombly, 1995, p. 44) (e.g. housekeeping, laundry, shopping etc).

Activity limitation and participation restrictions
The focus for occupational therapists is thus activity/occupation and when it comes to clinical praxis, activity limitation is central and the impact of environmental and social factors is emphasised. The complexity of activity and activity limitations is stressed in the World Health Organization classification *International Classification of Functioning, Disability and Health* (ICIDH-2). The aim of the classification is to present a uniform language and framework for description of health and health-related diseases and it has been in development since 1980.

The ICIDH-2 includes two main parts: (1) functioning and disability and (2) contextual factors. Functioning and disability includes body and activities and participation components, and contextual factors include environmental and personal factors. A person's disability is conceived as an interaction between health conditions (diseases, disorders, etc) and contextual factors. Activity, defined as the execution of a task or action by an individual, interacts with the components (body and activities/participation) and the factors (environmental and personal). The health condition (disease or disorder), body functions (physiological and psychological), body structure (anatomical parts), environmental (physical, social and attitudinal) and personal (background of life and living) factors and participation (in life situations) all influence the individual's ability to perform activities (WHO, 2000). The ICIDH-2 emphasises the close relationship between activities in daily life and health, including participation in meaningful activity in the areas of self-care, work, leisure and community life (McLauglin Gray, 2001).

Activity limitations and/or participation restrictions have been described as common consequences of a variety of diseases or symptoms e.g. rheumatoid arthritis (Nordenskiöld, 1996), stroke (Löfgren, 1999), fibromyalgia (Henriksson, 1995) and long-term pain (Blyth et al, 2001).

Pain

The International Association for the Study of Pain (IASP) (Merskey, 1979) defines pain as *"An unpleasant sensory and emotional experience associated with actual or potential tissue damage, or described in terms of such damage. Note: Pain is always subjective... "*(p. 250). Pain can be described in several respects like *duration* e.g. acute, chronic, long-term (Andersson et al., 1993; Brattberg, 1988,1989; Merskey, 1979), *type* e.g. nociceptive, neurogenic, psychogenic, idiophatic (SOS 1997), *diagnosis* (Adolfsson & Råstam, 1992), *intensity levels* e.g. discomfort, marked pain and considerable pain (Brattberg, 1988; 1989), *localisation* e.g. head, neck, shoulders/arms etc. (Brattberg, 1989), *character* e.g. burning, aching, gnawing (Gaston-Johansson, 1985), *affective/emotional* aspects e.g. irritation, sleeplessness, stress feelings (Gaston-Johansson, 1985; SOS, 1997) and *behaviour* e.g. chronic pain syndrome, coping (SOS, 1997).

Acute pain overpasses to chronic when normal healing has past (Bonica, 1953) but since "normal healing" may vary, it is suggested by the IASP to consider pain chronic after a 3-month duration (Merskey, 1996). However, the notion chronic pain gives the impression of an incurable and everlasting state, which is not always true why the notion of long-term pain has been suggested to be preferable (SOS, 1997).

Prevalence of long-term/recurrent pain

Prevalence studies of long-term pain (3 to >6 months) in two parts of Sweden showed rates of 46-66 % (Andersson et al, 1993; Brattberg et al, 1989) but no incidence rates were reported. These impairment-studies showed that pain increased with age up to 59-64 years, and that the most common area of pain was neck-shoulder and lower back. Studies in Australia (Blyth et al, 2001), Canada (Crook et al, 1984), Germany (Chrubasik et al, 1998), Denmark (Andersen Worm-Pedersen, 1987), and the USA (Sternbach, 1986) have given prevalence rates of chronic pain of between 11 and 31 %. The results of pain prevalence studies seem to depend on the definitions and instruments used (Brattberg et al, 1989, Linton & Ryberg, 2000).

Long-term pain in a gender perspective

The mentioned Swedish prevalence studies showed no gender differences concerning pain prevalence (Andersson et al, 1993). However, the ones performed in Germany (Chrubasik et al, 1998) and Australia (Blyth et al, 2001) demonstrated that pain was more frequent among women than among men. Results from the Australian study (Blyth et al, 2001) showed that pain had an impact on daily occupations especially among young women. Gender-related variables influencing pain are depression particularly among younger women and older men (Averill et al, 1996), a substantial history of trauma especially among men (Spertus et al, 1999), and body image distortion and fatigue among women (Novy et al, 1996). Females have been rated by social insurance officers as having a higher potential than men to benefit from rehabilitation (Jensen et al, 2000), but contradictory results were reported by the National Swedish Social Insurance Board (1999). The latter report showed that men were assessed to have a higher probability to return to work although both sexes had the same social history and reason for sick-leave (neck/back pain). Gender was the strongest determinant of whether a person on sick-leave got rehabilitation or early sickness pension. Men more often received rehabilitation and women early sickness pension. In a study in northern Sweden, it was concluded that men's behaviour and goals were consistent with the structures of the rehabilitation system, which may be an explanation of why men were favoured in the rehabilitation process (Ahlgren & Hammarström, 2000).

One study of chronic pain has been found concerning health care needs and use of health care services performed with a gender perspective. Women were reported to use more specific health care services than men, which was partly explained by more psychological needs in the former group (Weir et al, 1996).

Long term-pain and health care utilization

Among health care institutions in Sweden, the most frequently reported provider of care for pain patients was primary health care (Andersson et al, 1999a). Between 1987 and 1996, the number of health care visits in primary care of individuals with pain-related diagnoses increased by almost 25 % (Andersson et al, 1999b). There appears to be no study concerning what specific health care staffs pain sufferers visit. The frequency of health care visits among spinal pain sufferers in Sweden was re-ported to be an average of 3 during a 12-month period (Linton et al, 1998) and 3.5 in a replication study (Linton & Ryberg, 2000). However, the distribution of the con-sumption of resources was highly skewed as a small number of patients (6 %) ac-counted for more than 50 % of the costs (Linton & Ryberg, 2000). Engel et al (1996) denoted 2 or more follow-up visits as a high use of back-pain related primary care.

Health care utilization has been found to be influenced by high pain intensity, ag-ing and socio-economic level (blue-collar-workers, farmers and employees reported chronic pain more often than white-collar workers) (Andersson et al, 1999a; Engel et al, 1996), by depression (Andersson et al, 1999a; Engel et al, 1996; Zitman et al, 1992), history of sexual/physical abuse (Alexander et al, 1998), frequent low-back pain, health beliefs and socio-cultural factors (Szpalski et al, 1995). Interventions with a focus on activity limitations (e.g. behavioural treatments) have been suggested as a possible way to reduce health-care costs and utilization (Engel et al, 1996). No study has been found of persons with long-term/recurrent pain concerning the extent to which health care needs influence health care utilization. However, Ward (1997) reported that more frequent visits to rheumatologists among rheumatoid arthritis pa-tients were associated with improvements in pain and functional disability.

Pain management

Treatment of pain conditions may be categorized in (1) aetiological, (2) symptomatic, and (3) rehabilitative (SOS, 1997). Two critical analyses of the literature concerning evidence-based interventions for persons suffering from long-term pain showed that behavioural treatment, multidisciplinary treatment (Karjalainen et al, 2000; SBU, 2000), stress management, education combined with physical training (SBU, 2000), and biofeedback and reactivation (Karjalainen et al, 2000) seemed to be important components of treatment for this patient category.

Occupational therapy in pain management

Occupational therapy in pain management is one of a number of disciplines in the field of rehabilitation. Occupational therapists are often represented in the multi-disciplinary team (Bellner, 1998; Strong, 1996; Turk & Okifuji, 1998). On basis of occupational therapy literature, Strong (1996) concluded that the overall aim of oc-cupational therapists in pain management is *"maximizing the patient's functional status and control over her life, and minimizing the patients' loss of role and associ-ated competences... through specific techniques and engagement in purposeful ac-tivities."* (p. 50) Additional goals proposed for occupational therapy in pain man-agement concern various perspectives such as *general* (health promotion), *individual pain-management* (e.g. improve pain-control, increase pain-tolerance), *performance* (e.g. improve performance in home maintenance), *regain/maintain functions* (e.g. maintain/re-establish competence and/or roles) and *psychological* (e.g. improve self-esteem) (Table 1).

Areas of concern for occupational therapy have been suggested to include per-sonal self-care, housework, work and leisure (Caruso & Chan, 1986; Scudds & Solomon, 1995; Strong; 1986; 1987; 1996; 1998). Psychosocial and environmental factors are additional areas of concern in the discipline (Gibson & Strong, 1998; Phil-ips et al, 1997; Scudds & Solomon, 1995).

Table 1: Goals of occupational therapy interventions in pain management proposed in references focusing on occupational therapy

Goals	References
Health promotion	Fast, 1995; O'Hara, 1992
Improve performance in home maintenance	Phillips, Bruehl & Harden, 1997
Improve posture and body mechanics	Phillips, Bruehl & Harden, 1997
Improve quality of life	Carruthers, 1997; Giles & Allen, 1986
Increase independence	Fishman Borelli, Warfield, 1986; Strong, 1989; Strong, Ashton & Large, 1994; Ventura & Flinn-Wagner 1997
Increase own responsibility	Strong, 1989
Increase pain control	Strong, 1989
Increase pain-tolerance	Heck, 1988
Increase self-esteem	Fishman Borelli, Warfield, 1986; Klayman-Callahan, 1993; Scudds & Solomon, 1995; Strong, 1989
Maintain/re-establish competence	Fishman Borelli, Warfield, 1986; Johnson, 1984; Strong, 1989; Strong, Ashton & Large, 1994
Maintain/re-establish roles	Johnson, 1984; Klayman-Callahan, 1993; Phillips, Bruehl & Harden, 1997; Scudds & Solomon, 1995; Strong, 1989; Strong, Ashton & Large, 1994; Ventura & Flinn-Wagner 1997
Maximise function	Fast, 1995; Johnson, 1984; Scudds & Solomon, 1995; Strong, 1989; Strong, Ashton & Large, 1994
Reduce pain	Fishman Borelli, Warfield, 1986; McCormack, 1988
Regain balance in daily occupations	Blakeney, 1984; Johnson, 1984
Regain control	Carruthers, 1997; Johnson, 1984; Strong, 1989; Strong, Ashton & Large, 1994
Restore self-efficacy	Scudds & Solomon, 1995

As previously mentioned, occupational therapists focus on patients' activity limitations and/or participation restrictions. The <u>interventions</u> suggested in the literature for use in occupational therapy pain management demonstrates a wide range of broadly defined treatments, that may be used by several members in the rehabilitation team. The suggested interventions have various foci such as *initial assessments and planning* (e.g. assessment task of performance/activity analysis, attitudes assessment, goal setting), *occupational performance* (e.g. work hardening, ergonomics, energy conservation), *external adaptation* (e.g. assistive devices, splinting) or *educational perspectives* (e.g. pain education, back school). The interventions may also be labelled by the way activities were used, i.e. with a *behavioural* perspective (e.g. ergonomics, activity tolerance) or as a *tool* (e.g. arts and crafts, purposeful activities). Some of the interventions were described by several authors, for example "work conditioning", while others were mentioned in a small number of articles only (e.g. "assessment/ modify attitudes", "pain reporting") (Table 2).

Table 2: Occupational therapy interventions in pain management proposed in the literature

Intervention	References
Activity tolerance/endurance training	Caruso & Chan, 1986; Flower et al, 1981; Giles & Allen, 1986; Klayman-Callahan, 1993; Phillips, Bruehl & Harden, 1997; Scudds & Solomon, 1995; Ventura & Flinn-Wagner, 1997
Adaptation of environment	Herbert & Rochman, 1998
Arts and crafts	Carruthers, 1997; Ventura & Flinn-Wagner, 1997
Assessment task performance/ activity analysis	Blakeney, 1984; Klayman-Callahan, 1993
Attitudes assessment	Strong, 1998
Attitudes modify	Strong, 1998
Assistive devices	Giles & Allen, 1986; Scudds & Solomon, 1995; Strong, 1986
Back school	Klayman-Callahan, 1993
Biofeedback, TNS	Giles & Allen, 1986
Body mechanics training	Aja, 1991; Caruso & Chan, 1986; Flower et al, 1981; Klayman-Callahan, 1993; Phillips, Bruehl & Harden, 1997; Strong, 1986
Counselling	Scudds & Solomon, 1995; Strong, 1984; Strong, 1986; Strong, 1987
Energy conservation	Giles & Allen, 1986
Ergonomics	Caruso & Chan, 1986; Herbert & Rochman, 1998; Klayman-Callahan, 1993
Goal setting (interaction patient and therapist)	Herbert & Rochman, 1998; Klayman-Callahan, 1993; Strong 1992; Wiskin, 1997
Group activities/counselling	Carruthers, 1997; Herbert & Rochman, 1998; O'Hara, 1992; Scudds & Solomon, 1995; Strong, 1986
Joint protection	Giles & Allen, 1986
Pain education	Carruthers, 1997; Flower et al, 1981; Klayman-Callahan, 1993; Scudds & Solomon, 1995; Strong, 1984; Strong, 1998; Wiskin, 1997
Pain reporting	Flower et al, 1981
Purposeful activities	Heck, 1988; McCormack, 1988; Scudds & Solomon, 1995
Relaxation techniques	Flower et al, 1981; Giles & Allen, 1986; Herbert & Rochman, 1998; Johnson, 1984; McCormack, 1988; Strong, 1984; Strong, 1986; Strong, 1991; Ventura & Flinn-Wagner, 1997; Wiskin, 1997
Splinting	Aja, 1991; Strong, 1986
Stress management	Aja, 1991; Flower et al, 1981; Herbert & Rochman, 1998; Strong, 1986; Strong, 1987; Ventura & Flinn-Wagner, 1997
Work conditioning and work hardening	Aja, 1991; Caruso & Chan, 1986; Flower et al, 1981; Gibson & Strong, 1998; Giles & Allen, 1986; Klayman-Callahan, 1993; O'Hara, 1992; Phillips, Bruehl & Harden, 1997; Scudds & Solomon, 1995; Strong, 1986; Strong, 1987; Velozo, 1993; Ventura & Flinn-Wagner, 1997

Objectives of the present thesis

In times of limited financial resources and with the aim to distinguish persons who have the most benefit from health care interventions, needs assessment has been stated as a priority issue. Few studies with a needs assessment perspective have been performed in occupational therapy/rehabilitation and none has been found concerning persons with long-term/recurrent pain.

The prevalence and impact of self-perceived activity limitations/participation restrictions due to long-term/recurrent pain among persons aged 18-58 years have not been fully explored in Sweden. Such a study would be of interest to explore the need for occupational therapy interventions. If occupational therapy interventions to meet these needs were known, an initial step could be taken towards Swedish guidelines concerning occupational therapy for the target population.

AIMS

The overall aims of the present thesis are to describe (1) needs for occupational therapy among persons with self-perceived activity limitations and/or participation restrictions due to long-term/recurrent pain, and (2) treatment interventions in occupational therapy to meet demonstrated needs. The Liss' (1990) model for assessing health care needs is used to structure the purposes described below.

1. *To establish the actual state of self-perceived activity limitations/participation restrictions due to pain among persons aged 18-58 years with long-term/recurrent pain.*

   1.1. Establish the prevalence (Study I) and incidence (Study II) of self-perceived activity limitations/participation restrictions due to pain (the Study Group).

   1.2. Investigate differences between age groups concerning prevalence of self-perceived activity limitations/participation restrictions due to pain (Study I).

   1.3. Investigate differences between the Study Group and those without pain concerning demography, occupations in daily life and work (Study II).

   1.4. Describe the Study Group concerning, pain, coping and health care utilization (including institutions visited and treatments recommended or arranged on their own initiative) (Studies II, V).

   1.5. Investigate gender differences in the Study Group concerning pain, occupations in daily life, work and health care utilization (including institutions visited and treatments recommended or arranged on their own initiative) (Studies II, V).

   1.6. Describe persons in the Study Group with need of rehabilitation/occupational therapy with respect to demographic, pain, coping, work and treatment variables (Study III).

   1.7. Describe persons in the Study Group who had participated in occupational therapy with respect to demographic, pain, coping and, work variables and occupations in daily life (Study III).

1.8. Identify specific pain-related characteristics that may be used to distinguish patients who have the most benefit from occupational therapy (Studies I-III, V).

1.9. Investigate differences between groups of low and high health care consumers concerning pain-related characteristics (Study V).

2. *Settle the goals of occupational therapy for persons aged 18-58 years with self-perceived activity limitations/participation restrictions due to pain.*

   2.1. Describe the goals suggested by Swedish occupational therapists to be used for treatment interventions in pain management (Study IV).

   2.2. Describe the needs for occupational therapy for patients with long-term pain assessed by Swedish occupational therapists (Study IV) and as self-perceived by the Study Group (Study V).

   2.3. Investigate differences between groups of low and high health care consumers concerning self-perceived needs for occupational therapy (Study V).

3. *Determine the object of need for persons aged 18-58 years with self-perceived activity limitations/participation restrictions due to pain.*

   3.1. Describe the areas and interventions that Swedish occupational therapists suggest/offer in pain management (Study IV).

   3.2. Investigate relationships between assessed needs for occupational therapy and interventions in occupational therapy suggested/offered by Swedish occupational therapists (Study IV).

METHODS

An overview of the periods of data collection, designs, participants, methods for data collection, and statistical analysis in Studies I-V is presented in Table 3.

Table 3: Overview of the methods and subjects in Studies I-V

	I	II	III	IV	V
Period of data collection	May – October 1998	January – April 1999	January – April 1999	April – August 2000	October – November 2000
Design	Correlational	Comparative	Correlational	Correlational	Correlational
Participants	Swedish population aged 18-58 years	1) Persons with long-term/ recurrent pain 2) Persons with no pain	1) Persons with long-term/ recurrent pain 2) Occupational therapists	Occupational therapists	1) Persons with long-term/ recurrent pain
Number of participants	7,706	1) 1,305 2) 117	1) 914 2) 30	109	1) 443
Method of data collection	Questionnaires	Questionnaires	Questionnaires	Questionnaires	Questionnaires
Statistical analyses	Chi ^{2} Spearman rho	Chi ^{2} Students t-test Principal Component Analysis Cronbach's alpha coefficient	Chi ^{2} Spearman rho Principal Component Analysis Cronbach's alpha coefficient Logistic regression analysis	Chi ^{2} Principal Component Analysis Cronbach's alpha coefficient	Chi ^{2} Students t-test Principal Component Analysis Cronbach's alpha coefficient

Subjects

Four samples were included in the studies;

1. a sample of the Swedish general population ages 18-58 years (Study I),
2. persons with activity limitations/participation restrictions due to long term/recurrent pain (Studies I-III and V),
3. persons with no current or previous pain (Study II),
4. occupational therapists working in pain management (Studies III, IV).

Persons with/without pain (Studies I – III and V)

A randomly selected sample (n = 10,000) from the Swedish general population, ages 18-58 years, constituted the Study Group in Studies I-III and V. The sample size was based upon a power analysis made by Statistics Sweden using an expected rate of 200 persons with long-term or recurrent pain who should have participated in occupational therapy. The analysis was based on the reported Swedish prevalence rates for long-term pain of 46-66 % (Andersson et al, 1993; Brattberg et a., 1989) and the number of occupational therapists registered in the Swedish Union for Occupational Therapists (n = 7,000).

Persons with pain were of two categories, those who presently had and those who previously had had long-term/recurrent pain. Persons without pain included those who had no current or previous experience of long-term/recurrent pain. The inclusion of the subjects in Studies I-III and V is illustrated in Figure 2, and background data (gender, age, native country, civil status, housing, education level, long-term pain, recurrent pain and long-term and recurrent pain) for respondents with and without long-term/recurrent pain are presented in Table 4.

Occupational therapists (Studies III – IV)

The majority of occupational therapists were randomly selected from the register of the Swedish Union for Occupational Therapists. Some were recruited from an interest group focusing on pain management and from a pain course for occupational therapists. All answers provided by participants were anonymous.

In Study III, 47 of the 62 occupational therapists from the interest group and/or pain course were contacted. Thirty (64 %) responded and were willing to participate in the study.

In Study IV, fifty percent (n=425) of the occupational therapists that had reported themselves as working in primary health care in the Swedish Union for Occupational Therapists were contacted with a postal inquiry of participation. After two reminders, 85 occupational therapists (20 %) had responded. To investigate the poor response rate, 164 were contacted by telephone in alphabetic order. Ninety-four persons

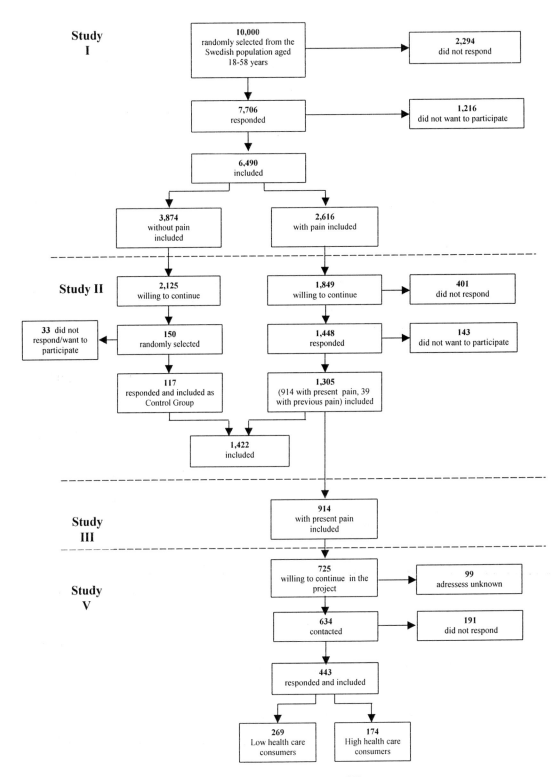

Figure 2: Subject inclusion (presented in frequencies) in Studies I-III and V.

Table 4: Background data and frequencies of long-term and/or recurrent pain, presented in percent for persons participating in Studies I-III and V. LHC = Low Health Care consumers; HHC = High Health Care consumers

		I		II		III	V	
							With pain	
		With pain	*Without pain*	*With pain*	*Without pain*	*With pain*	*LHC*	*HHC*
Frequency (n)		2,616	3,874	1,305	117	914	269	174
Gender	Men	42.5	51.0	38.1	47.9	37.0	43.1	27.6
	Women	57.5	49.0	61.9	52.1	63.0	56.9	72.4
Age-groups	1940-1949	-	-	29.9	37.8	31.7	41.2	46.0
born	1950-1959	-	-	30.0	20.5	31.2	32.6	28.2
	1960-1969	-	-	23.8	20.5	23.0	17.2	17.8
	1970-1979	-	-	14.0	15.4	12.3	8.6	6.3
	1980	-	-	2.4	3.4	1.9	0.4	1.7
Native country	Sweden	-	-	85.0	92.3	82	-	-
	Other	-	-	13.0	6.8	16	-	-
Civil status	Single	-	-	18.9	19.7	18.2	-	-
	Married/cohabit	-	-	69.9	70.9	69.7	-	-
	Widow/widower	-	-	1.8	1.7	1.8	-	-
	Divorced	-	-	7.7	7.7	8.5	-	-
Housing	Owned house	-	-	50.0	60.7	49.2	-	-
	Rented house	-	-	4.8	2.6	4.7	-	-
	Flat – co-operative	-	-	11.9	15.4	12.3	-	-
	Flat – with right of tenancy	-	-	27.3	16.2	27.6	-	-
	Other arrangement	-	-	5.0	0	4.7	-	-
Education level	< 7 years	-	-	12.1	4.3	14.4	9.2	13.3
	7-9 years	-	-	17.3	12.8	17.3	19.2	18.2
	10-12 years	-	-	31.8	26.5	30.5	36.8	41.2
	> 13 years	-	-	27.4	48.7	25.9	34.8	27.3
Long-term pain		19.4		23.5		23.5		
Recurrent pain		38.0		31.5		31.5		
Long and recurrent pain		42.6		45.0		45.0		

- = Not assessed

could be reached by 1, 2 or 3 telephone calls made on different occasions. Of the contacted occupational therapists, 11 had already responded, 25 did not work with this patient category, 27 did not want to participate (e.g. lack of time, not working now) and 31 answered that they should reply after this reminder. Fourteen actually did respond, giving a total of 99 respondents (23 %) of which 32 reported that they did not work with this patient category.

Of the 62 occupational therapists, working in and particularly interested in pain management, 42 (69 %) responded. The final sample consisted of 109 therapists (Study IV).

Information to respondents and definitions used

Together with a postal inquiry concerning participation in the study(-ies), the respondents received information about each specific study and an information folder about the research project as a whole (performed and planned studies). The respondents were informed that activity limitations and/or participation restrictions as a consequence of pain were a main condition to fulfil the inclusion term of pain. The information included the definitions described below.

Activity limitation and/or participation restriction (WHO, 1998) was defined in terms of the consequences of pain: *"The consequences of pain should limit the performance, fully or partly, of those daily activities (e.g. employment, housework or other wanted or obligatory occupations) that would have been performed if pain had not existed"* (Studies I-V).

Pain was defined according to the recommendations of the International Association for the Study of Pain (Merskey, 1979): *"experience of pain is subjective and can occur as a result of sickness or tissue damage. Pain can also occur in the absence of obvious sickness or damage. Pain can be experienced in different ways, e.g. as dull burning, pressing, splitting, sharp etc"* (Studies I-V).

Long-term pain was defined as persistent pain with a duration of more than three months and regularly recurrent pain as pain recurring more than once a month and lasting for more than 24 hours (Studies I-V).

Pain intensity was defined at three levels; (1) pain (recently occurring pain or discomfort in some part of the body); (2) marked pain (pain comparable with stiffness after exercise or more intense which affects and bothers one substantially or more); and (3) severe pain (pain comparable with sprained ankle, pulled muscle, tonsillitis which affects and bothers one to a very high degree or more) (SOS, 1997) (Studies II-III).

Need for occupational therapy was interpreted to exist when problems/activity limitations were reported for which remedy could be expected using occupational therapy treatment interventions (Studies IV-V).

Measures

An overview of the questionnaires with data levels and respondents is given in Table 5. The items in the questionnaires "Pain and occupations" including treatment options from the Swedish Council on Technology Assessment in Health Care (SBU, 1991), the "Occupational Therapy Needs Assessment–Pain" (OTNA-P) and "Pain-related characteristics" are presented in Appendices 1-3. Lists of areas and interventions of concern in occupational therapy are presented in Appendix 2:2.

Table 5: The questionnaires used in Studies I-V presented with data levels and respondents

Questionnaires	Study	Respondents	Data levels	See also
Prevalence of pain and activity limitations	I	Swedish population aged 18-58 years	Nominal	
Pain and occupations	II, III	Persons with and without long-term/ recurrent pain	Nominal Ordinal	Table 6 Appendix 1:1 Appendix 1:2
List of treatment options from the Swedish Council on Technology Assessment in Health Care	II	Persons with long-term/ recurrent pain	Nominal	Appendix 1:3
Occupational Therapy Needs Assessment – Pain (OTNA-P) plus a list of areas and interventions of concern in occupational therapy	IV	Occupational therapists	Nominal	Appendix 2:1 Appendix 2:2
Occupational Therapy Needs Assessment – Pain Patient (OTNA-PP)	V	Persons with long-term/ recurrent pain	Nominal Ordinal	
Pain-related characteristics	V	Persons with long-term/ recurrent pain	Ordinal	Appendix 3
Consumption of care	V	Persons with long-term/ recurrent pain	Ordinal	

Results of Principal Component Analyses of items of "Pain and occupations" (emotional/affective effects of pain, coping and treatments), the OTNA-P and the list of suggested areas and interventions in occupational therapy (attached to OTNA-P) are presented in Appendices 1 and 2.

Prevalence of pain and activity limitations (Study I)

The questionnaire, including the main conditions of pain (i.e. activity limitations/ participation restrictions as a consequence of pain, pain duration >3 months or recurrent pain = more than once a month and more than 24 hours per occasion) consisted of five questions (1) *"Do you have long-term pain?"*, (2) *"Do you have recurrent pain?"*, (3) *"Have you had long-term pain?"*, (4)*" Have you had recurrent pain?"*, and (5) *"Would you consider participating in further studies in this project?"*. The description of the inclusion criteria of self-perceived activity limitations/participation restrictions and pain together with the above questions was used to estimate the prevalence of self-perceived activity limitations/participation restrictions due to long-term/recurrent pain. The scale used was a dichotomous yes/no response-format.

Pain and occupations (Studies II-III)

To examine dimensions of long-term/recurrent pain and the impact of pain on performance of daily occupations (e.g. personal care, work and leisure) as perceived by the respondents, a questionnaire "Occupation and pain" was constructed and used in Studies II and III, including 142 items (Appendix 1:1). It was constructed on the basis of a literature review (Table 6) and included items concerning *demographic* variables (items 1-6), *pain* (i.e. duration, items 7-10; diagnosis, items 11-12; intensity, item 13; localisation, items 14-23; character, items 24-32; and affective/emotional effects; items 33-51), *occupations in daily life* (basic ADL (items 52-53, 57) and intermediate ADL (items 54-56, 58-62), satisfaction with health (item 63), sick leave days (item 64), social activity (items 65-68), work performance (items 69-75), *coping* (items 76-81), and *work* (social support, items 82-86; psychological job demands, items 87-91; and decision latitude, items 92-97). In addition, there were questions about undergone *treatment* (items 98-128), *care institutions* visited (items 128-133) and *hospital/care staff* consulted (items 134-142). Occupations in daily life were assessed by parts of the instrument the "Functional Status Questionnaire" (Jette et al, 1986; Rubenstein et al, 1989; Söderback et al, 1993), and coping by parts of the

24

Table 6: The questionnaire "Pain and occupations" used in Studies II and III with Cronbach's Alpha Coefficients

Purpose of the assessment	Alpha coefficients		Variables	References	No. of items	Data level	Scale range / No. of response options
	Study II	Study III					
Demography			Gender	Crook et al, 1984 SBU, 1991 Brattberg et al, 1988	1	Nominal	2
			Age	Brattberg et al, 1988, 1989	1	Scale	18-58
			Native country	Adolfsson & Råstam, 1992	1	Nominal	2
			Civil status	SOS, 1994 Gaston-Johansson, 1985	1	Nominal	4
			Education (years)	SOS, 1994 Gaston-Johansson, 1985	1	Ordinal	4
			Housing	SOS, 1994	1	Nominal	5
Pain	0.83	0.84	Duration	Brattberg et al, 1988,1989 Andersson et al, 1993 Merskey, 1979	4	Ordinal	2
			Diagnosis	Adolfsson & Råstam, 1992	2	Nominal	2
			Intensity	Brattberg et al, 1988, 1989	1	Ordinal	3
			Localisation	Brattberg et al, 1988	10	Nominal	12
			Character	Gaston-Johansson, 1985	9	Nominal	11
			Affective / emotional	SOS, 1997 Gaston-Johansson, 1985	19	Ordinal	4
Occupations in daily life[1]	0.82	0.77	Basic ADL	Jette et al, 1986	3	Ordinal	5
			Intermediate ADL	Jette et al, 1986	8	Ordinal	5
			Social activity	Jette et al, 1986	4	Ordinal	5/6
			Work performance	Jette et al, 1986	7	Ordinal	3/4
			Sick leave days	Jette et al, 1986	1	Scale	0-365
Coping	0.88	0.65	Strategies	Lazarus, 1991 Ahlström, 1994	6	Ordinal	4
Work[2]	0.77	0.75	Social support	Karasek, 1979 Karasek & Theorell 1990	5	Ordinal	4
			Psychological job demands	Karasek, 1979 Karasek & Theorell 1990	5	Ordinal	4
			Decision latitude	Karasek, 1979 Karasek & Theorell 1990	6	Ordinal	4
Treatment	0.84	0.84		SBU, 1991 SOS, 1997	31	Nominal	3
Care institutions	0.82			SOS, 1997	6	Ordinal	4
Hospital/care staff	0.55	0.58		SOS, 1997	9	Ordinal	4

[1] The Functional Status Questionnaire [2] The Swedish version of the demand/control questionnaire

instrument the "Assessment of Problem-focused Coping" (Ahlström, 1994; Tollén & Ahlström, 1998). Work-related variables were assessed by a Swedish modified version of the "Job Content Questionnaire" (Theorell et al, 1993) derived from the "demand/control/support model" (Karasek, 1979; Karasek & Theorell, 1990).

The Functional Status Questionnaire (FSQ) was developed in the USA as a screening instrument for disability including psychological, social and physical functioning. The FSQ includes the subscales: basic ADL (e.g. personal self-care), intermediate ADL (e.g. shopping), social activity (e.g. visit friends), work performance (e.g. hours of work), mental health (e.g. mood) and quality of interaction (e.g. feelings towards others) (Jette et al, 1986). Each subscale ranges between 0 and 100. Warning zones have been developed for each subscale, based on expert consensus statements for identification of important functional disabilities (Jette et al, 1986; Rubenstein et al, 1989). These can be used to identify persons who might need rehabilitation/occupational therapy (Söderback et al, 1993). The FSQ has been used in Sweden and found to be a useful instrument to detect difficulties in daily occupations among chronic back pain patients (Söderback et al, 1993). The subscales (warning-zones in brackets) basic (0-89) and intermediate ADL (0-72), social activity (0-78) and work performance (0-75) were included in the questionnaire "Pain and occupations" for assessment of the dimensions of occupations in daily life. The Swedish translation was made by Söderback et al (1993).

The instrument Assessment of Problem-focused Coping (APC) was developed for assessing coping strategies in daily occupations (Ahlström 1994; Tollén & Ahlström, 1998). The instrument is based on Lazarus and Folkman's definition of coping (Lazarus 1991; Lazarus and Folkman, 1984) and has been used in Sweden to assess coping strategies among persons with muscular dystrophy and other types of muscular weakness (Nätterlund & Ahlström, 1999). The APC includes 32 basic activities classified in five general occupational forms (personal care, home management, leisure, mobility and transportation, and work). The response alternatives cover problems (e.g. doing activity without or with problems), problem-focused coping (e.g. perform activity in a new/different way; perform activity by employing technical aids) and satisfaction (e.g. function well; does not function very well but I accept it) (Nätterlund, 2001; Nätterlund & Ahlström, 1999). Only the response alternative of problem-focused coping was used here. The items were constructed as questions and included in the questionnaire "Pain and occupations" to identify general ways of coping in daily occupations e.g. to perform the task in an alternative way.

A Swedish modified version (Theorell et al, 1991,1993) of the "Demand/Control Questionnaire" (Karasek, 1979; Karasek and Theorell, 1990) originally based on the Job Content Questionnaire/Quality Employment Survey-questionnaire (Karasek et al, 1998) and the demand/control/support model (Karasek, 1979; Karasek and Theorell, 1990), was included in the questionnaire "Pain and Occupation". The aim was to assess job strain in the dimensions psychological demands (five questions), decision latitude (six questions) and social support (five questions) that could influence job-related illness. Analysis of those dimensions allows prediction of workers' well-being and health (Karasek et al, 1998). The Job Content Questionnaire has been widely used (Karasek et al, 1998) e.g. in studies concerning musculoskeletal symptoms (Skov et al 1996) and pain (van Oel et al, 1995).

The list of treatment options for back pain were taken from the classification of treatments of The Swedish Council on Technology Assessment in Health Care (SBU, 1991). This list of treatments was a result of a critical review concerning causes, diagnostics and treatments of back pain. The back pain treatments represented those most frequently used in Sweden.

Occupational Therapy Needs Assessment – Pain (OTNA-P) (Study IV)
The instrument OTNA-P was developed to elucidate needs of occupational therapy interventions for persons with long-term pain (Appendix 2:1). The questionnaire was based on an existing instrument, the "Occupational Therapy Needs Assessment" (OTNA), constructed for assessment of cancer patients' need of occupational therapy interventions (Söderback & Hammersly Paulsson, 1997; Söderback et al, 2000). The OTNA has been tested for internal consistency with Cronbach's Alpha (α) Coefficients on two occasions, resulting in α coefficients of 0.92 (Söderback & Hammersly Paulsson, 1997) and 0.87-0.89 (Söderback et al, 2000) for the occupational therapy factor. Content validity was determined through literature search and construct validity by factor analysis (Söderback et al, 2000). The OTNA-P contents were based on literature reviews (Studies II, IV) and it was intended for use by occupational therapists or other health care professionals, when assessing need for occupational therapy. The questionnaire includes eighteen items of which one concerns the location of

27

pain (nominal scale; yes/no: item 1b) and one is a qualitative assessment of the patient's main activity limitation (item 2). The remaining sixteen items, rated on a nominal-scale (yes/no: items 3-18) were based on considerations of areas, goals and interventions proposed in the literature.

In addition, a list was included concerning <u>areas and interventions in occupational therapy</u>, based on a literature review of the same topics. The occupational therapists selected from the list of interventions which one(s) she/he had suggested/offered to a specific patient during the previous month and in what area the offered intervention(s) would be classified. Each intervention and area was defined. The occupational therapists were asked to define the goal(s) of each of the interventions. All items employed a yes/no format. The OTNA-P items and the list of areas and interventions are presented in Appendix 2 together with the results of performed Principal Component Analyses.

Occupational Therapy Needs Assessment – Pain Patient (OTNA-PP) (Study V)

The questionnaire OTNA-PP is based on the OTNA-P and is intended for use by persons with long-term/recurrent pain to assess their self-perceived needs of occupational therapy interventions (Appendix 2:1). The OTNA-PP includes nineteen items of which one concerned the localisation of pain (item 1b) and one if the respondent has previously been referred to occupational therapy or not (item 19), both using a yes/no format. Of the remaining seventeen items, based on areas, goals and interventions in occupational therapy, two (items 3-4) have a yes/no format and fifteen (items 4-18) are rated on an ordinal scale (never, sometimes [1-2 times/week], often [3-4 times/week] and always [5-7 times/week]). Compared to the OTNA-P, two additional items were included: *"Do you perform daily activities you wish or have to do despite pain?"* and *"Have you previously been referred to occupational therapy due to pain?"*. One question from the OTNA-P was deleted (item 2: *"What activity limitation would you consider be the main problem for the patient?"*)

Pain-related characteristics

This questionnaire was used to assess specific pain-related characteristics for persons with self-perceived activity limitations due to long-term/recurrent pain. It is based on results from Studies I-III. The items concerned fourteen characteristics of which eleven were rated on an ordinal scale and three used a yes/no format (Table 7).

Table 7: Pain-related characteristics included in the questionnaire used in Study V

Characteristics	Response options	Results from Study-(ies)
Gender	man; women	I, II, III
Age	18-19; 20-29; 30-39; 40-49; 50-59 years	I, II, III
Education	< 7; 7-9; 10-12; > 13 years	III
Previous long-term/recurrent pain	yes; no	I
Previous sick-leave due to pain	yes; no	II
Searing/aching/gnawing pain	never; sometimes(1-2 times/week); often (3-4 times/week); always (5-7 times/week)	II, III
Pain in shoulders/lower back	as above	II, III
Easily tired	as above	III
Restlessness	as above	II
Depressed	as above	II
Irresolution	as above	III
Difficulties to perform daily activities	as above	II
Repeated work task	as above	III
Changes needed at work place due to pain	none; some; few; many; don't have a job	III

Consumption of care (Study V)

This questionnaire included items concerned with what health care staff the respondents had consulted as a consequence of long-term/recurrent pain, how often and the time for the consultation(s) during the previous year. The response options were divided in 2-month periods, and respondents could mark whether they had visited health care professionals (physicians, nurses, occupational therapists, welfare officers, psychologists, physiotherapists, chiropractors and other health care givers) 1-2 times or $\geq$ 3 times in each 2-month period and for each health care professional. This questionnaire was used to collect data on visits to health care professionals and to identify low and high health care consumers.

Procedures

Study I

The subjects were contacted by a postal inquiry of participation including a question-naire, the "Prevalence of pain and activity limitations". The respondents could reply either by a pre-paid envelope or by a free phone telephone answering service. The data collection, including three reminders, resulted in a response rate of 71 %, (n=7,706) of which 6,490 could be included in the study (Figure 2).

Study II

The Study I respondents with self-perceived activity limitations/participation restrictions due to pain, who were willing to continue in the research project (n=1,849), received a postal questionnaire ("Pain and occupations"; Appendix 1:1). After two reminders, the response rate was 78 % and 1,305 persons were included. The Study Group of persons with pain consisted of those who had present long-term/recurrent pain (n=914) and those who previously had had such pain (n=391). A Control Group without pain (n=150) was randomly selected from the sample without pain in Study I. Inclusion criteria were no current or previous pain and willingness to continue in further studies. A total of 117 persons (78 %) were included in this manner (Figure 2). The Control Group completed the same questionnaire as the Study Group concerning demographic variables, occupations in daily life and work.

Study III

Respondents with activity limitations/participation restrictions due to present long-term/recurrent pain in Study II (n =914) were included.

The factor "ergonomics" (ergonomic counselling, ergonomic practical training, change of work environment, change of work organization) derived from the Principal Component Analysis of the questionnaire "Pain and occupations" (Appendix 1:2; factor 3) was used as the dependent variable "participated in occupational therapy" in the logistic regression analysis. To verify this choice, a list of treatments options in the classification of treatments by The Swedish Council on Technology Assessment in Health Care (SBU) (1991) was sent to occupational therapists (n = 47) working with pain patients. The purpose was to determine to what extent the treatment options

30

were considered by occupational therapists as treatments to offer pain patients. Thirty occupational therapists responded (64 %). The most frequently marked were: "ergonomic counselling" (100 %); "change of work organisation" (93.3 %); "work hardening" (90.0 %); "ergonomic practical education" (76.6 %); "back school" (73.3 %); "change of the work – environment"(70.0 %) and "bio-feed-back" (70.0 %). Four of these treatment options ("ergonomic counselling", "change of work organisation", "ergonomic practical education", and "change of the work-environment") were identified as belonging to the factor "ergonomics".

Study IV

Occupational therapists (n = 109) were asked to use the instrument OTNA-P to assess one or more of their patients aged 18-58 years with activity limitations/participation restrictions due to long-term pain with diagnoses classified as musculoskeletal and connective tissue diseases (in codes M06.P–M96.P, Swedish version of International Classification of Diseases and Related Health Problems, Tenth Revision, The Swedish National Board of Health and Welfare, 1997). The assessed patients should either be under occupational therapy treatment or ones that had finished treatment during the previous month. The assessment concerned the patients' need for occupational therapy interventions, using the OTNA-P and a list of interventions and goals. If such needs were demonstrated, the occupational therapists stated what interventions she/he had suggested to the patient including the area in which it was categorised (e.g. personal care, work, leisure) as well as the goal(s) of the intervention. No further instructions were given for the assessments. The occupational therapists assessed a total of 113 patients.

Study V

Subjects with self-perceived activity limitations/participation restrictions due to long term/recurrent pain, willing to continue in the research project (n = 725) were mailed a set of postal questionnaires including the OTNA-PP, "Consumption of care" and the questionnaire concerned with specific pain-related characteristics. Ninety-nine questionnaires were returned with unknown addresses giving a final sample of 634 of which, after one reminder, 69 % (n = 443) responded (Figure 2). The sample was divided into a Low Health Care consumers group (LHC) (n = 269) and a High Health Care consumers group (HHC) (n=174). This division was made on the basis of whether the respondents had visited health care professionals (physicians, nurses, occupational therapists, welfare officers, psychologists, chiropractors or other health care givers) 4 or fewer times during the previous year (LHC) or more than 4 times (HHC). The cut-off score of four times was based on previous studies with 3-3.5 health care visits as an average or high health care utilization (Engel et al, 1996; Linton et al, 1998; Linton & Ryberg, 2000).

Statistical methods

The specific statistical analysis methods used are presented in Table 3 and they are described in detail in the respective studies. The Statistical Package for the Social Sciences (SPSS) was used (1998, 1999). Level of significance was set at $p \leq 0.05$ in all studies. Frequency rates were used for overall description of the data.

Differences between genders, age-classes and between groups who had had long-term/recurrent pain and those who had pain at present were analysed by Chi-square statistics (Study I).

Differences between the Study Group (persons with long-term/recurrent pain) and the Control Group (persons without present or previous pain) were analysed by Chi-square statistics (nominal data: e.g. gender, housing, work variables), or Students t-test (continuous data: e.g. education, occupations in daily life assessed by the FSQ) respectively. In the Study Group, differences between genders were investigated by Chi-square statistics (nominal data: e.g. pain variables, occupations in daily life assessed by the FSQ, work variables, sick-leave, treatment and health care staff visited) (Study II).

The computation of the incidence rate was based upon data from the Control Group (i.e. persons who had reported no present or previous pain in Study I) and the number of respondents who had developed pain during the interval between their participation in Study I and Study II (8 month interval) (Riegelman & Hirsch, 1996) (Study II).

Logistic regression analysis was used in Study III to investigate associations between independent variables (e.g. demographics, pain, coping, work) and two dependent variables: (1) need of rehabilitation/occupational therapy and (2) participation in occupational therapy. Need of rehabilitation/occupational therapy was determined on the basis of the results of the FSQ. Respondents were considered to have need for rehabilitation/occupational therapy if they scored in stated warnings zones in one or more of the FSQ subscales (number of respondents at or in warning-zones: Basic ADL = 351; Intermediate ADL = 253; Social Activity = 351; Work Performance = 854; Total [in one or more warning zones] = 886). Participation in occupational therapy was determined on the basis of whether the participants had received treatments in the factor "ergonomics"(Appendix 1:2, factor 3) (n = 315) or not. A data reduction procedure was used to limit the number of predictive variables. Univariate analyses (chi-square-tests, Spearman rho) were performed to find variables (demographic, pain, coping, occupations in daily life) associated with the dependent variables. Items concerning affective/emotional effects of pain, treatment options and coping strategies showed significant intercorrelations and were included in Principal Component Analysis (Varimax rotation) (Appendix 1:2). From each component, the independent variable that showed the strongest association with the dependent variable was selected for inclusion in the logistic regression analyses. In the first analysis (need of rehabilitation/occupational therapy), 15 predictive variables were chosen and in the second (participation in occupational therapy), 16 (Table 8). All predictive variables were entered in the equation simultaneously, as there were no specific hypotheses about their importance or order (Study III).

Principal Component Analyses (Varimax rotation) were used for data reduction and Cronbach alpha was used for analysing the internal consistency of the generated factors (Studies II-V).

Differences between high and Low health care consumers were investigated by Chi-square statistics and the Students t-test (Study V).

Table 8: Independent variables included in logistic regression analysis of prediction of need for rehabilitation/occupational therapy (analysis 1) and participation in occupational therapy (analysis 2) (n=914) (Study III)

Analysis	Factor/sub-scales	Item	Appendix 1:1 item no
1, 2	**Demographic**	gender	1
1, 2		age	2
1		native country	3
1		years of education	5
	Pain		
1, 2	*location*	shoulders	16
2		hips	22
2		lower back	21
2	*character*	burning pain	24
1		searing pain	25
1		gnawing pain	27
2		aching pain	29
2	*affective/emotional effect*	depressed	33
1, 2		easily tired	39
2		sensitive	43
1		irresolution	48
	Occupations in daily life[1]		
2	*Basic ADL*	ability to perform personal self-care	52
2	*Intermediate ADL*	ability to perform housework	58
2	*Social activities*	ability to take care of others	67
2	*Work performance*	ability to perform ordinary work tasks but with some changes due to health	74
2	*Satisfaction with health*		63
1	**Coping**[2]	avoiding tasks	80
1		using technical aids	77
2		use of tricks and/or compensated ways when performing tasks	76
2		performs tasks partly	81
	Work[3]		
1		supporting workmates	85
1		learn new things at work	92
1		same work tasks over and over again	95
1		control over work task performance	96

[1] The Functional Status Questionnaire; [2] The Assessment of Problem-focused Coping; [3] The Swedish version of the demand/control questionnaire

Ethical considerations

All studies were approved by the Research Ethics Committee at the Faculty of Medicine, Uppsala University.

All respondents received information about the study, the project as a whole (performed and planned studies) and a short description of occupational therapy in pain management. They were also informed that all information gained would be treated with confidentiality and that they could terminate their participation without any explanation at any time they wished.

RESULTS

The actual state of self-perceived activity limitations/participation restrictions due to long-term/recurrent pain

Prevalence and incidence of self-perceived activity limitations/participation restrictions due to long-term/recurrent pain (Studies I and II)

The prevalence of self-perceived activity limitations/participation restrictions due to long-term/recurrent pain was found to be 26 % with an incidence of 0.07.

The frequency of pain reports increased significantly with age and the highest levels were reported by women with long-term and/or recurrent pain aged 40-58 years (26.7–27.3 %).

Differences between the group with pain and those without pain (Study II)

Demographic data: The respondents with self-perceived activity limitations/participation restrictions due to long-term/recurrent pain (Study Group) did not differ concerning age, native country or civil status from those without pain (Control Group). The Study Group had fewer years of education (mean = 11.7 years) than the Control Group (mean=12.9) (t =4.6; df =1,263; p<0.001) and there were more owned houses (Chi^2=4.9; df=1; p=0.026) and co-operative apartments (Chi^2=5.5; df =1; p=0.019) in the Control Group.

Performance of daily occupations assessed by the Functional Status Questionnaire (FSQ) showed that the majority (93.1 %) in the Study Group were unable to perform employed work which was significantly higher than in the Control Group (24.8 %) (t=17.0; df=1,420; p<0.001). More than a third (38.9 %) in the Study Group had difficulties to perform basic ADL but fewer (21.5 %) reported problems with intermediate ADL. Nobody in the Control Group reported having problems with intermediate ADL and very few with basic ADL (0.9 %). Significant differences were found between the groups (Intermediate ADL: t=8.9; df=1,420; p<0.001; Basic ADL: t=6.5; df=1,420; p<0.001). Social activity did not differ between those with and without pain. In the Study Group, sick leave during the previous year was reported by 55.7 %

(mean=43 days) which was significantly higher than the Control Group (mean=12 days) (t=3.8; df=1,029; p<0.001). Over half of the respondents (53.3–57.6 %) experienced working conditions that fell within one or more of the risk zones assessed by the demand/decision/support questionnaire. Persons in the Control Group reported higher frequencies of poor social support measured separately and in combination with lack of control (Chi^2=4.3; df=1; p=0.039). These findings indicate that the Study Group had significantly more problems than the Controls for all daily occupations (work performance, basic and intermediate ADL) but the Control Group experienced poorer social support than did the Study Group.

Perceptions of pain, coping strategies and health care utilization (Studies II, V)
Descriptive pain variables showed that of those who had received a diagnosis (67.2 %), a majority (78 %) had musculoskeletal and connective tissue diseases (codes 710-739). The localizations were most frequently in the shoulder/arm (50 %) and lower back (52 %) and the most common characteristics of pain were searing (43.2 %) and aching (60.4 %). Emotional/affective effects of pain were reported by a majority of respondents: 1)"restlessness" (90.1 %), 2) "depressed" (86.4 %), 3) "anxious" (80.6 %), 4) "insufficient" (70.4 %) and 5) "dispirited" (68.0 %). A majority (82.3 %) of the respondents with pain had also had long-term/recurrent pain earlier.

Between 62.5 and 82.4 % of the Study Group used one or more coping strategies (i.e. avoid the task [82.4%], technical aids [80.8 %], compensating by tricks or stratagems [62.5 %]).

Primary health care was the most frequently visited health care institution. The reported range of health care visits was between 0 and 46 (m=5.58, Md=2, SD=7.48). One third (32.2 %) of the respondents reported no visit and one tenth (10.2 %) reported one visit to a health care professional during the previous year. The distribution showed that 60.5 % had visited a health care professional 4 or fewer times. Among health care staff, physicians had the highest frequency of visits (74 %) followed by physiotherapists (55.3 %) and chiropractors (30.4 %). About one fifth (19.7 %) had met a nurse and every tenth (11 %) an occupational therapist from whom they had received treatment. The five most frequent treatments recommended in health care according to self-report were medicines (59.6 %), muscular stretching (42.9 %), physical activation at home (35.4 %), rest/confinement to bed (34.4 %) and massage (29.8 %). Treatments that respondents had arranged themselves were (the five highest frequencies): massage (25.8 %), medicines (23.2 %), physical activation at home (22.3 %), manipulation of joints (20.3 %) and rest/confinement to bed (20.0 %). These results indicate that musculoskeletal pain in shoulders/lower back is accompanied by a high level of perceived emotional/affective effects. It is also accompanied by a high frequency of health care visits, most often to primary health care physicians and physiotherapists.

Gender differences (Studies II, V)

The overall frequency of self-perceived activity limitations/participation restrictions due to pain was higher among women than among men (Chi^2=4.3; df=1; p=0.038), while there were no differences in duration, intensity or diagnosis. More women reported <u>pain</u> located to head (Chi^2=31.0; df=1; p<0.001), neck (Chi^2=31.0; df=1; p<0.001), shoulder/arms (Chi^2=48.0; df=1; p<0.001), abdomen (Chi^2=4.5; df=1; p=0.033), pelvis (Chi^2=16.7; df=1; p<0.001), upper back (Chi^2=31.4; df=1; p<0.001), and hips (Chi^2=15.7; df=1; p<0.001). Women were also more affected than men by insufficiency (Chi^2=27.0; df=1; p<0.001) and depression (Chi^2=45.4; df=1; p<0.001) and they were more dispirited (Chi^2=48.1; df=1; p<0.001). The character of pain differed between genders showing that burning (Chi^2=12.4; df=1; p<0.001), spasmodic (Chi^2=8.8; df=1; p=0.003), aching (Chi^2=31.4; df=1; p<0.001), sore (Chi^2=39.5; df=1; p<0.001) and tense pain (Chi^2=26.0; df=1; p<0.001) occurred more frequently among women than men.

Equal difficulties to perform <u>occupations in daily life</u> were reported by men and women in three of the four FSQ subscales. However, women reported more problems in performing intermediate ADL (e.g. shopping, house-work, laundry) than did men (Chi^2=15.8; df=1; p<0.001).

Concerning stress-related ill health at <u>work,</u> women reported higher job demands than men (Chi^2=6.0; df=1; p=0.014). However, more men than women perceived lack of control (Chi^2=18.9; df=1; p<0.001) and poor social support (Chi^2=14.1; df=1;

p=0.001). More women reported long sick-periods (>3 months) as compared to men ($Chi^2=7.2$; df=1; p=0.007).

No gender differences were found concerning visits to <u>health care institutions,</u> concerning how often clinics were visited or the kinds of clinics visited. Women reported more frequent visits to physiotherapists ($Chi^2=11.8$; df=1; p=0.001), occupational therapists ($Chi^2=18.0$; df=1; p<0.001), psychologists ($Chi^2=5.7$; df=1; p=0.017) and welfare officers ($Chi^2=14.1$; df=1; p<0.001), while men more frequently visited nurses ($Chi^2=4.7$; df=1; p=0.030) compared to women. Women generally tried more varied types of treatments than men, who underwent more surgery ($Chi^2=11.8$; df=1; p=0.001) including elective surgery ($Chi^2=4.5$; df=1; p=0.033) and joint manipulations ($Chi^2=6.9$; df=1; p=0.009). The treatment variables categorized as "ergonomics" ($Chi^2=20.0$; df=4; p<0.001) and "psychological support" ($Chi^2=12.6$; df=3; p=0.006) were more often used by women than by men.

These findings show a predominance of higher frequencies reported by women concerning the prevalence of self-perceived activity-limitations/participation restrictions due to long-term/recurrent pain and affective/emotional effects of pain. Women also had more difficulties with intermediate ADL, perceived higher job demands and had longer sick leave compared to men. Men perceived poorer social support than did women. Women visited more frequently various health care staff and generally tried more varied type of treatments compared to men.

Predictive variables indicating need for rehabilitation/occupational therapy (Study III)

Fifteen independent variables (Table 8) were included in the logistic analysis predicting the dependent variable need of rehabilitation/occupational therapy based on the FSQ. Those who had scored in the FSQ warning-zones were considered to have need of rehabilitation/occupational therapy.

Only one predictive variable was related to the outcome variable need of rehabilitation/occupational therapy. The variable "irresolution" predicted the outcome with an odds rate (OR) of 2.96 (p<0.05; 95 % CI=1.19–7.38). Irresolution refers to difficulties to make decisions.

When the FSQ subscales basic ADL, intermediate ADL, social activity, and work performance were used separately as dependent variables, several predictive relationships were identified. "Irresolution" and "gnawing pain" were predictive of all subscales but the strongest predictor differed between scales. Perceiving "searing pain" had more than twice as high odds ratio for having *basic ADL* problems compared to those without "searing" pain (p<0.001; OR=2.40; 95 % CI=1.82-3.16). The variable "gender" with an odds ratio of 0.52 indicated that women were twice as likely as men to have problems with *intermediate ADL* (p<0.001; 95 % CI=0.37-0.74). Feelings of "irresolution" were predictive of problems with *intermediate ADL* (p<0.001; OR=3.38; 95 % CI=2.45-4.67), *social activity* (p<0.001; OR=2.94; 95 % CI=2.18-3.93) and *work performance* (p<0.001; OR=3.24; 95 % CI=1.72-6.11). These results suggest that perceptions of "irresolution", "gnawing and/or searing pain" and "gender" (women) are the strongest predictive variables for need of rehabilitation/occupational therapy.

Variables predictive of participation in occupational therapy (Study III)

Participation in occupational therapy was used as dependent variable and those who had received "ergonomic" treatments (ergonomic counseling, ergonomic training, change of work environment or work organization; Appendix 1:2, factor 3) were considered to have participated in occupational therapy. Sixteen independent variables (Table 8) were included in the logistic analysis predicting the dependent variable.

Five variables were predictive of participation in occupational therapy. The strongest was whether one "used tricks and/or compensated ways to perform tasks". If this coping strategy was used, the odds were almost 2.5 that the person had participated in occupational therapy (p<0.001; OR=2.45; 95 % CI=1.76-3.42). "Pain in shoulders" had an odds ratio of nearly 2 (p< 0.001; OR=1.97; 95 % CI=1.45-2.68), "lower back pain" 1.74 (p<0.001; 95 % CI=1.28-2.36) and "aching pain" had an odds ratio of 1.64 (p<0.001; 95 % CI=1.19-2.26). Finally, the predictive variable "changes made at work due to health conditions" had an odds ratio of 1.45 for participation in occupational therapy (p<0.001; 95 % CI=1.25-1.68). These findings indicate that use of the coping-strategy "used tricks and/or compensated ways to perform tasks" and shoulder/lower back pain of aching character are the strongest predictors of whether a person has participated in occupational therapy or not.

Pain-related characteristics (Studies I-III, V)

Fourteen specific pain-related characteristics of persons with self-perceived activity limitations due to long-term/recurrent pain were found in Studies I-III reflecting demographics, pain (character, location, affective/emotional aspects) and occupations in daily life (Table 9). Differences between Low Health Care consumers (LHC) and High Health Care consumers (HHC) were found for all items except age and education. There was a predominance of women in the HHC group (72.4 % women; 27.0 % men; Chi^2=10.8; df=1; p=0.001). Remaining characteristics were reported more frequently in the HHC-group with the greatest differences between the groups in "difficulties in performing daily occupations due to pain", "easily tired due to pain" and "feelings of irresolution".

Table 9: Specific pain-related characteristics of persons with self-perceived activity limitations due to long-term/recurrent (%). Differences between high and low health care consumers reflected by Chi^2 (Study V)

From Study	Characteristic		Whole group n = 443	Chi^2	p-value
I, II, III	Gender (men/women)		36.8 / 63.2	10.8	0.001
I, II, III	Age[1] (years)	18-19; 20-29; 30-39; 40-49; 50-58	0.9; 7.7; 17.4; 30.9; 43.1	4.1	ns
III	Education (years)	< 7; 7-9; 10-12; >13	10.8; 18.7; 38.6; 31.9	3.9	ns
II	Previous sick-leave due to pain		39.3	48.1[2]	<0.001
I	Previous long term/recurrent pain previously		76.4	20.1[2]	<0.001
II, III	Shoulder/low back pain		89.6	47.7	0.020
II, III	Searing/aching/gnawing pain		92.1	47.1	<0.001
II	Restlessness due to pain		69.5	52.1	<0.001
II	Depressed due to pain		79.4	42.3	<0.001
III	Feelings of irresolution due to pain		63.1	61.8	<0.001
III	Easily tired due to pain		86.3	63.6	<0.001
II	Difficulties in performing daily occupations due to pain		76.4	72.7	0.007
III	Repeated work tasks		86.9	15.6	0.004
III	Changes needed at workplace due to pain		68.7	36.7	<0.001

Chi^2, df = 3; [1]= df = 4; [2] = df = 1

The goals of occupational therapy

The goals of occupational therapy in pain management (Study IV)
Occupational therapists working in pain management reported that the most frequent goals of their interventions were to reduce pain (23 %), to support the patient to maintain/re-establish competence (13 %) and to improve performance in home maintenance (13 %).

Need for occupational therapy (Studies IV-V)
Occupational therapists assessed need for occupational therapy among patients with long-term pain with the Occupational Therapy Needs Assessment-Pain (OTNA-P) instrument. Needs/problems as limitations in activity performance were reported most frequently: i.e. the patient was assessed to "interrupt" (96.5 %), "to get more pain" (92.9 %) or "to give up performance of activity" (92.0%) and "to perform activities with more effort" (88.5%) (Table 10). Principal Component Analysis (Appendix 2:1) resulted in five categories of assessed needs/problems: (1) "need for education", (2) "needs due to limitations in activity performance", (3) "needs due to discouragement", (4) "need as an effect of dependency" and (5) "needs related to work".

The respondents with long-term/recurrent pain assessed their needs for occupational therapy with the OTNA-PP. The respondents reported the highest frequencies for the items: "temporal imbalance concerning rest/work/leisure" (91.1 %), "perform activities with more effort" (89.8 %), "tense/stressed when pain occurs" (89.0 %) and "interrupt performance of activities due to pain" (86.7 %) (Table 10). Principal Component Analysis (Appendix 2:1) resulted in four categories of needs/problems: (1) "need for education", (2) "needs due to limitations in activity performance", (3) "need to regain activities" and (4) "adjustment difficulties".

Significant differences between low and high health care consumers were found for all items with the greatest differences in "dependent on others", "stopped performing activities", "need of changes in home/workplace" and "difficulties with perceived expectations" (Table 10).

41

Table 10: Percent needs/problems assessed by occupational therapists (Study IV) and as self-perceived by persons with long-term/recurrent pain in total, and differences between Low Health Care consumers (LHC) and High Health Care consumers (HHC) (Study V)

Otna-P ques- tion	Needs/problems assessed	Assessed by			
		Occupational therapists $(n=109)$ (Study IV)	Persons with long-term/ recurrent pain (Study V)		
			Whole group $(n=443)$	Differences between LHC and HHC groups Chi²	p-value
3	Need of changes in home or at workplace	71.7	40.4	30.5[1]	<0.001
4	Need of support to regain activities	76.1	34.5	25.1[1]	<0.001
5	Need of more knowledge about pain	74.3	84.6	11.9	0.001
6	Difficulties to adjust to changes	77.0	84.8	27.6	<0.001
7	Dependent on others	83.2	63.9	59.7	<0.001
8	Tense/stressed	82.3	89.0	30.8	<0.001
9	Need to learn new ways to handle activities	84.1	65.4	35.8	<0.001
10	Stopped performing activities	86.7	67.2	66.5	<0.001
11	Temporal imbalance concerning rest/work/leisure	56.6	91.1	9.9	0.020
12	Deficient self-confidence	57.5	76.5	47.0	<0.001
13	More pain in activity	92.9	83.0	37.8	<0.001
14	Interrupt activities	96.5	86.7	59.7	<0.001
15	Give up activities	92.0	84.1	55.5	<0.001
16	Perform activities with more effort	92.0	89.8	58.5	<0.001
17	Would like to be at workplace during sick-leave	41.6	63.1	12.2	0.007
18	Difficulties with perceived expectations	71.7	67.9	52.6	<0.001

Chi²; df = 3; [1]= df = 1

Of the four items with the highest frequencies reported by occupational therapists and by persons with long-term/recurrent pain, two items were identical ("interrupt activities", "perform activities with more effort").

The Principal Component Analysis (Appendix 2:1) resulted in five factors of assessed needs in the occupational therapists' study (Study IV) and four in the study where persons with pain were respondents (Study V) (Table 11). The factors "needs due to limitations in activity performance" and "need for education" were found in both studies but the remaining factors were not fully consistent between the studies. "Needs due to limitations in activity performance" consisted of eight items in Study V of which five were the same in Study IV. The remaining three items were found in the factor "discouraged" ("stopped performing activities" and "deficient self-confidence") and as the single item "dependency" in Study IV. The factor "need for education" included four items in both studies of which three corresponded. Remaining factors did not correspond between the studies.

42

Table 11: The factor structure of the OTNA-P and OTNA-PP according to Principal Component Analyses from the occupational therapists' study (Study IV) and the study with persons with pain as respondents (Study V).

Factors from the OTNA-P (Study IV)	Factors from the OTNA-PP (Study V)
Needs due to limitations in activity performance	**Needs due to limitations in activity performance**
Interrupt performance of activities due to pain	Interrupt performance of activities due to pain
Give up activities due to pain	Give up activities due to pain
Perform activities with more effort	Perform activities with more effort
More pain in activity	More pain in activity
Difficulties with perceived expectations	Difficulties with perceived expectations
	Dependent of others
	Stopped performing activities
	Deficient self-confidence
Need for education	**Need for education**
Need of more knowledge about pain	Need of more knowledge about pain
Need to learn new ways to handle activities	Need to learn new ways to handle activities
Tense/stressed due to pain	Tense/stressed due to pain
Difficulties to adjust to changes	Would like to be at workplace during sick-leave
Discouraged	**Need to regain activities**
Need of support to regain activities	Need of support to regain activities
Stopped performing activities	Need of changes in home or at workplace
Deficient self-confidence	
Temporal imbalance concerning rest/work/leisure	**Adjustment difficulties**
	Temporal imbalance concerning rest/work/leisure
Dependency	Difficulties to adjust to changes
Dependent of others	
Work related needs	
Need of changes in home or at workplace	
Would like to be at workplace during sick-leave	

The object of need

Areas and interventions in occupational therapy in pain management (Study IV)

The <u>areas</u> of concern for occupational therapy interventions were housework (88.5 %), personal care (63.7), leisure (56.6 %), work (53.1), environmental factors (40.7 %) and psychosocial factors (26.5 %).

All the listed <u>interventions</u> suggested in available literature were considered by the occupational therapists as possible interventions in occupational therapy with persons with long-term pain. Interventions were reported with frequencies between 19.5 and 87.6 %. The Principal Component Analysis (Appendix 2:2) revealed six categories of interventions (range of frequencies for the included items in brackets): (1) "education and stress management" (19.5–65.5 %), (2) "behavioral interventions" (28.8–87.6 %), (3) "hand treatment" (38.9–44.2 %), (4) "group activities" (22.1–32.7 %), (5) "activity tolerance" (13.3–34.5 %), and (6) "external adaptations" (39.8–74.3 %). The most frequently suggested interventions were: "counseling" (87.6 %), "assessment of task performance/activity analysis" (80.5 %), "energy conservation" (74.3 %), and "assistive devices" (74.3 %). The respondents suggested an additional 22 interventions, ten of which could be categorized within the existing list. The remaining 12 interventions were classified either as "hand training" (9.7 %) (e.g. motion training) or "pain relieving treatment" (8.0 %) (e.g. paraffin-bath) and were not included in the factor analysis performed of the interventions suggested from the literature. The findings suggest that interventions focusing on "behavioral interventions", "external adaptations", and "education and stress management" were the most frequently reported for occupational therapy use in pain management.

The relationships between factors of needs/problems and suggested interventions in occupational therapy (Study IV)

Significant correlations were found between some of the factors derived from occupational therapists' assessment of patient needs/problems for occupational therapy and the factors derived from their suggested interventions (Table 12).

Table 12: Correlations (Spearman rho) between occupational therapists' assessment of patient needs/problems and their suggested interventions (n=114)

Needs/problems factors	Intervention factors					
	Education & stress management	Behavioral interventions	Hand treatment	Activity tolerance	External adaptation	Group activity
Need for education	0.28**	0.24**	-0.17	0.17	-0.00	0.07
Limitations in activity performance	0.09	0.12	0.13	0.12	0.14	-0.01
Discouraged	0.32**	0.28**	-0.18	0.22*	0.08	0.05
Dependency	-0.10	-0.14	-0.03	-0.02	0.13	-0.16*
Work related needs	-0.01	0.14	0.13	0.07	0.25**	0.03

* =p< 0.05; **= p<0.01

Correlations were found between, on one hand, the needs/problems factors "need for education" and "discouraged" and, on the other hand, the intervention factors "education & stress management" and "behavioral interventions". The factor "discouraged" also correlated with the intervention factor "activity tolerance". "Work related needs" correlated significantly with the factor "external adaptation". The factor "limitations in activity performance" did not correlate with any intervention factor.

The specific item "need for more knowledge about pain" correlated significantly with sixteen of the occupational therapy interventions of which thirteen were categorized in "education and stress management" or "behavioral interventions". Difficulties with "temporal imbalance" correlated with ten interventions, nine of them categorized in "education & stress management" or "behavioral interventions". The item "would like to be at workplace during sick-leave" correlated with eight interventions (Table 13).

Table 13: Specific needs/problems correlating with interventions suggested by occupational therapists (Chi^2, df=1)

Interventions suggested by occupational therapists		Needs/problems assessed with OTNA-P					
		More knowledge about pain		Temporal imbalance		Would like to be at workplace during sick-leave	
Factor	Item	Chi^2	p-value	Chi^2	p-value	Chi^2	p-value
Education & stress management	Pain education	17.35	0.000	4.85	0.028	4.71	0.030
	Attitudes modify	9.43	0.002	7.18	0.007		
	Bio-feed back/TNS	6.99	0.008				
	Goal setting	6.90	0.009	5.74	0.017	4.44	0.033
	Stress management	6.48	0.001	8.55	0.003	4.57	0.033
	Attitudes assessment	6.11	0.013				
	Relaxation techniques	4.04	0.045	5.29	0.021		
Behavioral interventions	Body mechanics training			7.40	0.007	7.39	0.007
	Work conditioning/ hardening	9.51	0.002	7.67	0.006	15.31	0.000
	Ergonomics	8.58	0.003				
	Assessment task performance/activity analysis	5.65	0.017	11.19	0.001	6.30	0.012
	Energy conservation	5.06	0.025	4.21	0.040	6.48	0.011
	Counseling	4.38	0.036				
Hand treatment	Splinting	5.60	0.018				
Group activity	Group counseling	4.04	0.045				
	Back school						
Activity tolerance	Activity tolerance/endurance training	6.48	0.011				
	Purposeful activity					4.57	0.033
External adaptation	Assistive devices			3.90	0.048		

"Purposeful activity" (included in the factor "activity tolerance") was suggested when patients were assessed to be discouraged ("give up activities" [$Chi^2 = 4.67$; df = 1; p= 0.031], "deficient confidence on own ability" [$Chi^2 = 6.83$; df =1; p= 0.009]), and when they "perform activities with more effort" ($Chi^2 = 4.33$; df = 1; p= 0.037), "would like to be at work-place during sick-leave "($Chi^2 = 4.57$; df = 1; p= 0.033) and "need of adaptation/changes in home or at work", ($Chi^2 = 5.83$; df = 1; p= 0.016).

These results indicate that needs/problems categorized in "need for education" and "discouraged" were frequently assessed by the occupational therapist that suggested interventions categorized in the factors "education and stress management" and "behavioral interventions" as appropriate to meet the needs.

DISCUSSION

Needs assessment defines the probable need for a service or a program (Soriano, 1995). Needs may be defined and measured in different ways and the main point is to find an appropriate set of methods relevant to the actual circumstances (Wilkin, 1993). In this thesis, needs assessment was performed with the purpose to describe the need for occupational therapy among persons aged 18-58 years, with self-perceived activity limitations/participation restrictions due to pain, and to describe treatment interventions in occupational therapy to meet these needs. Liss' conceptualisation of needs assessment in health care was employed as a structural scheme.

The actual state

The rates for prevalence (26 %) and incidence (0.07) (Studies I, II) indicate the extent of self-perceived activity limitations/participation restrictions due to long-term/recurrent pain in the Swedish population aged 18-58 years. The present results differ from previous Swedish studies (Anderson et al, 1993; Brattberg, 1989) with reported prevalence rates between 46 and 66 %. There are several possible reasons for these differences. The studies differ with regard to definitions of terms, instruments for data collection, perspectives (i.e. impairment versus activity limitations/participation restrictions), and sampling (Brattberg et al, 1989; Linton & Ryberg, 2000). In one of the former prevalence studies (Anderson et al, 1993), definitions of pain focused on constant or regular pain of several types (e.g. dull, burning, stabbing) and was limited to pain with a duration of 3 months or more. In Study I, similar definitions were used (pain duration >3 months, regularly recurrent, several types etc.). However, an important difference was that activity limitation as a consequence of pain was the main condition for inclusion in the present studies. Prevalence studies of pain with large, randomly selected nation-wide samples have, to my knowledge, not been performed previously in Sweden. However, a recently reported nation-wide general health survey (n=17,543) in Australia (Blyth et al, 2001) showed prevalence rates of chronic pain of 17.1 % for males and 20.0 % for women, most of them reporting some degree of interference with daily occupations due to pain. That study seems more comparable to Study I with respect to sampling and results than do the previous Swedish prevalence studies.

The respondents with pain had fewer years of education than those without pain (Table 4). A similar result has been reported in an earlier Swedish study (The National Swedish Social Insurance Board, 1999).

A majority of the respondents had problems with occupations in daily life, mainly at work. More than half of the sample was in some of the risk-zones for job-related illness. Women who suffered from pain had more difficulties than men with intermediate-ADL, which has previously been reported (Jensen et al, 1994; Johansson et al, 1999). This might be because women more often then men are responsible for housework (The Swedish National Board of Health and Welfare, 1997). The results suggest that men and women react differently to stress-factors at work. More women than men felt that work demands were on such levels that they may develop stress-related illness. It has been reported that women on sick-leave due to long-term pain still have full responsibility for housework (Johansson et al, 1999), which may impact on perceived demands on work. On the other hand, more men stated that they lacked the control they wished for and they experienced low control together with low social support at work. Karasek et al (1998) compared six populations from the United States, Canada, Netherlands and Japan (total n=16,601) concerning the demand/control/support model, and found gender differences in only one sample (U.S.; n = 6,053). Women in that sample reported higher frequencies of perceived psychological demands than men, which agree with the present findings. However, persons without pain reported higher levels than those with pain of social strains both privately (measured by FSQ "social activity) and at work (measured by the "Demand/Control Questionnaire").

The Study Group with pain included a majority of women (Study II: 61.9 %) with diagnoses of the musculoskeletal system. Pain was located mainly to the shoulders (50 %) and lower back (52 %) and seemed to increase with age, confirming previous pain-prevalence studies in Sweden (Andersson et al, 1993; Brattberg, 1989). Affective/emotional aspects of pain were reported by the majority of the respondents. Comparable findings were reported in the Australian study with a high level of psychological distress among respondents with chronic pain that interfered with daily occupations, especially among females (Blyth et al, 2001). In a literature review, Linton (2000) found that correlations between psychological factors and neck/back pain were frequently reported. Gender differences were shown in Study II with more women than men affected by insufficiency, dispiritedness and depression. Similar results were reported by Jensen et al (1994) who found higher levels of affective distress (mood, tension) among pain-suffering women compared to men.

Primary health care and physicians were reported as most often visited due to long-term/recurrent pain which is in line with previous findings by Andersson et al (1999 a; b). The most frequently used treatments were medicines, muscular stretching, physical activation at home, rest, confinement to bed, and massage. These results are comparable to those of a German study where oral medication, massage, exercise treatment, mudpack and heat treatment were the most frequently reported by patients with long-term pain (Chrubasik, et al, 1998). The treatments that persons with pain had been recommended or sought on own initiative differed between men and women. Men underwent more "traditional medical care" such as surgery, including elective surgery and joint manipulations than did women. Women tried more varied types of treatments such as psychological support, practical ergonomic training, relaxation and body awareness training, which could be categorized as "para-medical treatment". Women more often than men had met various health professionals, probably as an effect of seeking different treatments. These gender differences are similar to those of Weir et al (1996) who reported that men's pain was more often attributed to physiological causes in contrast to women's which was explained in part by psychological need and meaning.

Logistic regression analyses were used as an additional method to elucidate characteristics of persons with long-term/recurrent pain with need for occupational therapy (Study III). Associations were sought between a number of independent variables (demography, pain, coping, occupations in daily life, work and treatment) and the dependent variables need for rehabilitation/occupational therapy and participation in occupational therapy. Perception of "irresolution" was the strongest predictive variable for need for rehabilitation/occupational therapy followed by "gnawing and searing pain" and "gender" (women). "Use of tricks and/or compensated ways to perform tasks", "pain in shoulders/lower back" and "aching pain" were the strongest predictive variables for participation in occupational therapy. Women with gnawing/searing/aching pain in shoulders/lower back were frequently represented in the Study Group and the predictive variables derived from the logistic regression may therefore be an effect of this fact. The strongest predictive variable for need of rehabilitation/occupational therapy was perception of "irresolution", which may be classified as a depressive symptom (the American Psychiatric Association, 1994). Depressive symptoms have been reported to be related to pain and disability (Linton, 2000), which supports the results of the present study. Furthermore, it may partly explain why "irresolution" emerged as the strongest predictive variable. Those who had participated in occupational therapy more often used tricks and/compensated ways to perform task than those who had not participated. Occupational therapy, focusing on occupational performance, may have the effect on participants that they more frequently use tricks/compensated ways to perform tasks.

The identification of characteristics that may be used to distinguish patients who have the most benefit from specific health care interventions has been stated as a necessity demand (SOS, 1999). In Studies I-III, fourteen specific pain-related characteristics were identified in the Study Group (Table 9). Although gender, age and education may be criticized for being too general to be suggested as possible criteria, previous studies (Ahlgren & Hammarström, 2000; Jensen et al, 2000; The National Swedish Social Insurance Board, 1999) indicate that gender should not be neglected. It has been reported that gender was the strongest determinant of whether a person got rehabilitation or sick-pension. Men more often than women got rehabilitation and women more often early sickness-pension (The National Swedish Social Insurance Board, 1999). Socio-economic circumstances have been reported to have an impact on health (The Swedish National Board of Health and Welfare, 1997). Blue-collar workers and employees were reported to have higher frequencies of chronic pain than others (Andersson et al, 1993). The majority of specific pain-related characteristics found (Studies I-III) are supported by results reported in previous studies. Pain of searing/aching/gnawing character located in shoulder/low back pain has previously been reported as the most frequently demonstrated characteristics and pain-locations (e.g. Andersson et al, 1993; Brattberg, 1989; Gaston-Johansson, 1985; SOS, 1997). Depressive symptoms (e.g. restlessness, irresolution, easily tired, depression) are often described as related to long-term pain (e.g. Arnstein et al, 1999). Depressive symptoms have been reported to increase with a longer pain duration (Averill, 1996), and depression, anxiety, distress and related emotions have been found to be associated with pain and disability (Linton, 2000). It has also been shown that persons with pain-related disability (activity limitations) may become depressed (Arnstein et al, 1999). Difficulties in performing daily occupations due to pain have also been reported in previous research (e.g. Blyth et al, 2001; Henriksson, 1995).

High Health Care consumers (HHC) differed from those with Low Health Care consumption (LHC) concerning all pain-related characteristics except age and education with increased frequencies in the HHC group. Previous studies of health care consumption have reported that depression (e.g. Andersson et al, 1999a) and frequent low back pain (Szpalski et al, 1995) increase health care consumption, which is in line with the results of Study V.

The goals of occupational therapy

The occupational therapists reported (Study IV) that the most frequent goals of interventions used were to reduce pain and to support the patient to maintain/re-establish competence and improve performance in home maintenance. The goal "to reduce pain", most often reported by the occupational therapists, seems to focus on impairment rather than on activity/occupation. An activity perspective has been proposed as the current occupational therapy view (Björklund, 2000). This difference may be a result of the gap between clinical praxis and theory as discussed by several authors (e.g. Alsop, 1997; Rebeiro, 1998) or an illustration of current diversity in occupational therapy. The two other frequently suggested goals (maintain/re-establish competence and improve performance in home maintenance) represent an activity perspective. The goal "to reduce pain" may also be an expression of the expected result of an improved occupational performance. These examples of activity and impairment perspectives may have several reasons as mentioned above. In addition, it may be an illustration of various perspectives in a still developing profession (Lund & Andersson-Nordberg, 1998). It may also be an effect of the fact that occupational therapists, often working in a medical context, have adopted at least a partial impairment perspective in order to work in better congruence with other health care professionals.

In the assessment of needs for occupational therapy interventions by the occupational therapists for their patients (Study IV) and by persons with long-term/recurrent pain (Study V), a more homogenous pattern was found among the occupational therapists. Three of their four highest ratings were given to items in the factor "needs due to limitations in activity performance" while the respondents with pain had only one of their three most frequently stated needs in this factor. These differences may result from the fact that these are two groups with different characteristics. The occupational therapist group is more homogenous demographically and has a similar approach to pain management grounded in education and praxis. The group consisting of persons with long-term/recurrent pain is naturally more heterogeneous and no theory or praxis tie them together. The greatest diversity between the assessments of these groups was found for the item "temporal imbalance concerning rest/work/leisure". Respondents with pain gave this a very high priority (91.1 %) but the occupational therapists rated it of less importance (56.6 %). The term "temporal imbalance" was not defined in the instrument and may therefore have been interpreted in various ways. One interpretation could be an overall perception of lack of time, which probably would give high ratings in any investigated group. However, this does not explain the reported difference in ratings. It may result from the fact that the assessments were made of two independent groups of persons with long-term pain. However, needs as a consequence of temporal imbalance should be explored further in future studies.

The object of need

The occupational therapists suggested interventions that focus on increased knowledge of handling daily occupations. These interventions were categorized in six main factors of which "education and stress management", "behavioral interventions" and "activity tolerance" correspond with interventions found to be effective for treatment of long-term pain problems, i.e. behavioral treatment, stress management, and education combined with physical training and reactivation (Karjalainen et al, 2000; SBU, 2000). The suggested interventions are also compatible with the ICIDH-2 classification system, i.e. the body and activity and participation components and the contextual factors (environmental and personal). The interventions suggested by the occupational therapists focused mainly on activity and participation e.g. "assess task performance/activity analysis", "evaluate work and work hardening" although the body component was also represented by e.g. "splinting" and "joint protection". The environment factor may be illustrated by the occupational therapy interventions "adaptations of environment" and "assistive devices".

Some of the interventions suggested for pain management by occupational therapists are broadly defined, e.g. relaxation techniques, stress management, and use of biofeedback. In addition, they are offered by health care professionals other than occupational therapists, e.g. physiotherapists and psychologists. During its development, occupational therapy has been influenced by several sources and disciplines (e.g. philosophy, psychology, sociology, education) (Kielhofner, 1992; Reed & Sanderson, 1999), which may explain the overlapping arsenal of therapeutic interventions. Occupational therapists, often working in rehabilitation teams, may have various work tasks, depending on the specific team (Bellner, 1997). Thus, work tasks overlap in rehabilitation. The specific contribution of the occupational therapist would be the activity perspective (Björklund, 2000; Reed & Sanderson, 1999), using activity/occupation as a tool e.g. in ergonomic practical training in natural everyday environments: e.g. baking or doing the dishes in a kitchen, and activity/occupation as a goal for intervention e.g. maintaining/re-establishing competence to perform housework. The broadly defined goals and/or interventions used by occupational therapists may also be an effect of a lack of a unified professional terminology, especially in Sweden (FSA, 1983). However, there is an ongoing discussion about the concept of occupation within occupational therapy, in a theoretical (e.g. Persson et al, 2001) as well as an empirical perspective (e.g. Erlandsson & Eklund, 2001). A continuing, vital discussion and research seems urgent since an important task within occupational therapy is to continue the development of its unique identity. On the other hand, seeking for similarities and commonalities between rehabilitation disciplines may also be a profitable way to develop rehabilitation professionals.

The OTNA-P needs "need for education" and "discouraged" were frequently assessed by the occupational therapists who suggested interventions focusing on "education and stress management" and "behavioral interventions" to meet the needs. These findings seem logical in the sense that need for education should be met by interventions with educational purposes. Several authors in occupational therapy stress the therapeutic use of purposeful activities (e.g. Reed & Sanderson, 1999) but also for pain management (e.g. Scudds & Solomon, 1995). This standpoint is in line with the ICIDH-2 in which health includes participation in meaningful activities (McLaughlin Gray, 2001). Occupational therapists who stated that persons with pain were discouraged (i.e. "give up activities", "deficient confidence on own ability") or had work-related needs (i.e. "would like to be at workplace during sick-leave", "adaptation/changes at work/ home"), also suggested purposeful activities as one of the interventions. Historically, purposeful activity has been one of the main concepts within occupational therapy (Christiansen & Baum, 1997; Reed & Sanderson, 1999). This concept seems still to be of interest to occupational therapy in pain management.

The present thesis indicates that the Liss' model of health care needs with three recommended steps could be successfully employed as a structural scheme. The *actual state* of self-perceived activity limitations/participations restrictions due to long-term/recurrent pain among persons in ages 18-58 years was investigated from two perspectives. The first focused on the extent of the problem (e.g. prevalence and incidence rates) indicating considerable proportions of self-perceived activity limitation/participation restrictions due to long-term/recurrent pain. The second perspective focused on the health status of the studied sample (e.g. demographic data, occupations in daily life, aspects of pain, gender differences) resulting in fourteen specific pain-related characteristics for the investigated sample. The second step in Liss' model, to settle the *goal of health care*, was assessed by asking occupational therapists directly about their goals, and indirectly by assessing needs for occupational therapy using occupational therapists and persons with long-term/recurrent pain as respondents. Three main goals and two categories of needs were identified that corresponded between the groups. Goals, implicitly derived from assessed needs, may be "reduce limitations in activity performance" (needs due to limitations in activity performance) and "increase knowledge about how to handle effects of pain" (need for education). The final step, determine the *object of need*, was explored by stating the areas and interventions in occupational therapy that could meet the needs and thereby approach the goals. Six areas of concern for occupational therapy interventions were reported. Reported interventions were categorized in six factors.

Of the three recommended steps, the first and second step resulted in information about the respondents, indicating a difference between the actual state and the goal of health. The third step resulted in proposed areas and interventions to reach the goals. However, the actual effects of suggested interventions remain to be examined in future research.

Methodological considerations

When using correlational and comparative designs, two essential features should be considered thoroughly: sampling and measurement. Large samples, representative of the population should be used, and accurate multiple measurements should be performed of each subject (Brink & Wood, 1989).

Subjects and procedures

The studies are based on four samples of which a nation-wide, randomly selected sample was the foundation for Studies I-III and V. The size of that sample was based on a power analysis performed to achieve at least 200 persons with long-term/recurrent pain who had participated in occupational therapy. Estimates were based on known prevalence rates of long-term/recurrent pain (Andersson et al, 1993; Brattberg, 1989) and the current number of occupational therapists working in Sweden (n= 7,000). The power analysis indicated that 8,000 persons should be included in Study I. To secure at least 200 persons with visits to occupational therapists, an additional 2,000 persons were included. Study II showed that 139 persons reported visits to occupational therapists due to pain. The number of persons in Study V who had received occupational therapy was 315. The true number of persons who had participated in occupational therapy is probably in the 139-315 range. Response rates of 60 % are suggested as sufficient (Polit & Hungler, 1995). In the present studies, responses rates varied between 70.0 % and 78.3 %. In Study I, the distribution of responses across Swedish counties, gender and age was scrutinized. This showed that the response distribution corresponded well to the Swedish population in these respects. In Studies II and III, the predominance of women increased but no further analyses of non-participants were done. The higher frequencies of females in the pain-groups correspond to findings in other studies of pain (e.g. Blyth, 2001). The original sample was a stratified random selection from the Swedish population, which supports the external validity of the findings (Brink & Wood, 1989). In addition, the response distribution corresponded to the Swedish population, and the response frequencies were 70 % or more. This suggests that the samples are probably representative of persons with self-perceived activity limitations/participations restrictions due to long-term/recurrent pain in the ages 18 – 58 years.

The respondents with pain in Study V were divided into groups of low and high health care consumers, depending upon how often they had visited health care professionals due to pain during the previous year. The cut-off score was set to more than 4 visits for high health care consumers based on previous studies of health care utilization for spinal pain sufferers (Linton et al, 1998; Linton & Ryberg, 2000). However, this cut-off score might have been set too low, as the mean in Study V was 5.6 visits, but on the other hand, data were skewed (md= 2). Thus, the chosen cut-off score appears to be adequate.

The occupational therapists participating in Study IV were randomly selected from the Swedish Union for Occupational Therapists with a very poor response rate (23 %). This is why approximately 40 % of the occupational therapists were contacted. The main explanations for non-participation, "lack of time" and "do not want to participate", do not indicate that the results of the study would have been different if the non-participants had responded. However, the poor response rate calls for caution when interpreting the results. The response rate among the occupational therapists with a special interest in pain management, probably representing a more homogenous group, was 69 %. Their answers may give a reasonable representation of occupational therapists in pain management, while the other group of occupational therapists represents primary care. Pain patients most often visit primary health care (Andersson et al, 1999b; Study II) for which reason the latter group of occupational therapists would be of interest in this perspective. Responses were anonymous and the groups could not be identified at this stage of research. The results should thus be interpreted with caution due to the small sample size and the large proportion of non-responders. Maybe an alternative data collection method would had been preferable, e.g. focus groups and/or Delphi surveys with occupational therapists and other key informants working in pain management. These methods require fewer participants and a purposeful sampling of occupational therapists working in primary health care and/or of those who are particularly knowledgeable about the issue would have been possible (Polit & Hungler, 1995).

The questionnaires

The questionnaires used in the present thesis were constructed for the specific studies, as no existing instruments seemed to fulfill the demands of data collection considering the study aims.

In Study I, the main aim was to establish the prevalence of self-perceived activity limitations/participation restrictions for persons with long-term/recurrent pain of ages 18-58 years. Another aim was to derive a sample that could be included in further studies. The large sample size (n=10,000) and the offer of responding to a free phone telephone answering machine (earlier not used in research according to the largest telecom company in Sweden) necessitated that the number and length of questions be minimized. The questions were short (e.g. "Do you have long-term pain?") which might have biased the aim of the study, i.e. establishing a study group of person with long-term/recurrent pain with activity limitations/participation restrictions. The short questions with a focus solely on pain, may have resulted in inclusion of those who had long-term/recurrent pain but no activity limitations/participation restrictions. This may have contributed to a falsely estimated prevalence rate. To counteract this risk, thorough descriptions of the main conditions of the study were provided in the questionnaire. These descriptions included definitions of activity limitations, participation restrictions, long-term pain, recurrent pain and two examples illustrating long-term/recurrent pain in two perspectives. The first example described a person who had long-term pain but no activity limitations/participations restrictions, illustrating a person who would not be included in this study. The other person had long-term pain causing self-perceived activity limitations/participation restrictions who should therefore be included in the study. The results from Studies II-III and V showed that performing daily occupations, in one way or other, was problematic among all the participating respondents. This indicates that the possible biasing effect of the short questions in the Study I questionnaire can be considered as limited. Another consideration is the previously reported prevalence rates of 49-66 % (Andersson et al, 1993; Brattberg, 1989), which are nearly, or more than twice as high as in Study I. In those studies, the investigated group ranged between 25 and 84 years, with the highest numbers in the age range of 45-64 years, which is consistent to the findings in Study I. The differences between the prevalence studies previously performed (Andersson et al, 1993; Brattberg, 1989) and Study I seem to support the conclusion of limited bias due to the short items in the questionnaire. The options for completing the questionnaire – by mail or telephone – proved of less importance. The majority (88.5 %) responded by mail. This result is surprising, since it seems more convenient and less time consuming to respond by telephone, but the respondents choose the "traditional" mail method.

The questionnaire "Pain and Occupations" (Appendix 1:1) used in Studies II and III are based on literature reviews and included parts of previously used and tested instruments (the Functional Status Questionnaire, the Assessment of Problem Focused Coping and the Demand/Control Questionnaire). Only parts and not the complete instruments were included in order to limit the number of items. Cronbach´s Alpha Coefficient for the main variables (pain, occupations in daily life, coping, work, treatments, care institutions, hospital/care staff) showed levels between 0.55 and 0.88 which indicates almost (0.55) and acceptable (>0.60) internal consistency (Table 6). Coping is described as strategies to handle stressful situations (Lazarus, 1991, Lazarus & Folkman, 1984) and problem-focused coping as a way to handle the

the stress (Nätterlund, 2001). Coping was assessed by "Pain and Occupations" and parts of the instrument "Assessment of Problem-focused Coping", but it is not known whether the respondents perceived the problems as stressful. The answers may therefore represent problem-solving strategies rather than problem-focused coping strategies.

The questionnaires "Occupational Therapy Needs Assessment–Pain" (OTNA-P) and "Occupational Therapy Needs Assessment–Pain Patient" (OTNA-PP) employed in Studies IV-V were developed on the basis of an existing instrument ("Occupational Therapy Needs Assessment"), constructed and used for assessing needs for occupational therapy among cancer patients (Söderback & Hammersly-Paulsson, 1997; Söderback et al, 2000). The OTNA-P(P) was also based on literature reviews of pain and occupational therapy. Although the OTNA-P(P) was constructed on the basis of literature reviews, the items seem to be formulated too broadly to be specific for occupational therapy. The occupational therapy studies identified in the literature review were mostly of a descriptive character, and only two were randomized controlled studies (Heck, 1988; Strong, 1998). It is necessary to continue the development of the questionnaire so as to make the items of more direct relevance for occupational therapy.

Another debatable aspect of the OTNA-P(P) is the rationale for construction of the items. The most straightforward approach would be to construct an instrument that focused directly on needs, that is, to ask the respondents about their needs. This would probably elucidate perceived/expressed needs. However, problems with daily life tasks as a focus in occupational therapy often seem to be unresolved or unexpressed by clients and other health care professionals (Söderback & Hammersly-Paulsson, 1997). In addition, persons with activity limitations/participation restrictions often adapt to the situation (Nätterlund, 2001) and may accept circumstances, which could be improved if they were recognized. The OTNA-P(P) questions were constructed to discover aspects of activity limitations/participation restrictions including those not expressed directly in terms of needs. The items were therefore not formulated in a straightforward manner (e.g. "Do you need practical ergonomic education?"). Instead, they focused on difficulties from an activity perspective (e.g.

"Does it happen that you have to interrupt the performance of activities due to pain [e.g. work, hobbies, housework]?") The results obtained by the OTNA-P(P) indicate the appropriateness of the problem-focused approach, since the lowest frequencies were found for those items where a straightforward formulation was used (e.g. "need of changes in home or at workplace"). The low frequencies may of course reflect the actual state, that is, few participants needed changes in their home or at the work-place. On the other hand, the results may also reflect unrecognized needs, since the participants may not be aware of what changes are possible in their homes or at their workplaces.

Data analysis

The incidence-rate calculated in Study II was based on a small sample (n=117), for which reason this estimate should be considered with some caution.

The factor "ergonomics" (Appendix 1:2, factor 3) was used as a dependent variable, "participation in occupational therapy", in the logistic regression analysis in Study III. An alternative may have been to use the results from those who had reported visits to occupational therapists in the questionnaire "Pain and Occupations". The latter alternative was not chosen since a confusion among the respondents seemed to exist concerning if they had visited an occupational therapist or a physiotherapist. In the rehabilitation team, work tasks often overlap between professionals, particularly between occupational therapists and physiotherapists (Bellner, 1997). This may explain this confusion. The respondents received a short description of occupational therapy in the information folder. This may have contributed to the confusion as the described work tasks of an occupational therapist in the information folder, may actually have been administrated to the respondent by a physiotherapist. However, when analyzing the data with the alternative independent variable (reported participation in occupational therapy, n=139), significant results emerged. The strongest predictor was "pain in hips" with the odds of 2.52 (p=0.003; 95% CI=1.53-4.14) followed by "use of tricks and/or compensated ways to perform tasks" (p=0.005; OR=1.63; 95% CI=1.24-2.15). The strongest predictor, "pain in hips" did not emerge in the previous analyses. Patients with hip pain often visit occupational therapy for assistive devices, which may be an explanation of the present result. These results of analyses with two alternatives for "participation in occupational therapy" as dependent variables, indicates that "use of tricks and/or compensated ways to perform tasks" is a consistent predictor.

Another weakness of the OTNA-P and OTNA-PP is the different response options, the former using a yes/no format and the latter an ordinal scale. This limited the possibility of statistical analysis, as the factors from the Principal Components Analyses were not comparable.

SUMMARY OF FINDINGS

- The prevalence of self-perceived activity limitations/participation restrictions due to long-term/recurrent pain among persons in the age range 18-58 years, was found to be 26 % with an incidence of 0.07.

- Specific pain-related characteristics that may be used to distinguish persons who have the most benefit from specific health care interventions were identified. Fourteen characteristics of the Study Group were found. Demographic characteristics were female gender, in the ages between 40 and 58 years and fewer years of education than persons without pain. Pain in shoulders/lower back of searing/aching/gnawing character were the most frequently reported. A majority of the respondents reported depressive symptoms (irresolution/depression/restlessness/easily tired) and they had had previous sick-leave due to pain. Pain interfering with the performance of daily occupations, repeated work tasks and changes needed at work place due to pain were additional distinguishing variables. High health care consumers reported higher frequencies of all pain-related characteristics except age and education compared to low health care consumers.

- Women reported higher frequencies concerning prevalence of self-perceived activity limitations/participation restrictions due to long-term/recurrent pain and affective/emotional effects of pain. Women also had more difficulties with intermediate ADL, perceived higher job demands and had longer sick leave compared to men. Men perceived poorer social support than did women. Women visited more frequently various health care staff and generally tried more varied type of treatments compared to men.

- Predictive variables for need for rehabilitation/occupational therapy were perception of "irresolution", "gnawing and/or searing pain" and "gender" (women).

- A predictive variable indicating participation in occupational therapy was the use of the coping strategy "used tricks and/or compensated ways to perform tasks".

- According to the occupational therapists, the main goals for interventions in occupational therapy were to "reduce pain" and "maintain competence/improve performance of home maintenance". Goals, implicitly derived from assessed needs were "reduce limitations in activity performance" and "increase knowledge about how to handle effects of pain".

- Need for occupational therapy interventions categorized as "limitations in activity performance" (i.e. "interrupt/avoid to perform activities", "get more pain in activity", "perform activities with more effort", and "difficulties with perceived expectations") was the most frequent need/problem among pain patients according to occupational therapists. The persons with long-term/recurrent pain reported the highest frequencies of needs as a consequence of "temporal imbalance concerning rest/work/leisure" and "perform activities with more effort".

- Occupational therapy interventions could be categorized in six factors: "education and stress management", "behavioral interventions", "hand treatment", "group activity", "activity tolerance", and "external adaptations".

- Needs/problems categorized in "need for education" and "discouraged" were frequently assessed by the occupational therapist who suggested interventions categorized in the factors "education and stress management" and "behavioral interventions" as appropriate to meet the needs.

- High health care consumers reported more self-perceived needs than low health care consumers, mainly concerning interference with daily occupations.

Conclusions and suggestions for future research

The results of this thesis show that the prevalence of self-perceived activity limitations/participation restrictions due to long-term/recurrent pain is considerable among persons of ages 18-58 years. Needs/problems categorized as limitations in activity performance and temporal imbalance were frequently reported and interventions in occupational therapy to meet reported needs were suggested. High health care consumers reported needs/problems more frequently than did low health care consumers. This indicates an urgent area of research for occupational therapy.

However, the relationship between difficulties to perform occupations in daily life and need for occupational therapy has to be investigated in further studies. The OTNA-P(P) questionnaire may be helpful to assess need for occupational therapy but the instrument has to be developed further to be more specific to the profession. The outcomes of occupational therapy interventions have scarcely been examined. If the effects of occupational therapy interventions in pain management could be demonstrated, it would not only help to clarify the complex relationship between needs and interventions, but a development towards selection criteria for occupational therapy could also be initiated. The fourteen specific characteristics that were identified in this thesis may form the first step towards distinguishing persons who may benefit from occupational therapy. However, these characteristics should be scrutinized in the light of the effects of occupational therapy interventions. That is, if occupational therapy interventions have a positive effect on participants, some of these problems (e.g. depressive symptoms, difficulties in performing daily occupations) should be reduced.

ACKNOWLEDGEMENTS

I wish to express my gratitude to all persons who have supported and contributed to this work in different ways. I would like to express my warmest thanks to all of them. In particular, I am grateful to:

- *all persons* who were included in the studies, persons with or without pain, and occupational therapists. Without your contribution this work had not been possible,
- *Ingrid Söderback*, who has generously shared her scientific knowledge with me, for support and guidance in the scientific world,
- *Per-Olow Sjödén*, the head of the Section of Caring Science, for providing a most comprehensive doctoral education and for supervising me in the final stage of this work,
- *Gunnel Kristiansson*, Mälardalens University, who had confidence in me and the courage to employ me as doctoral candidate,
- *Birgitta Svall, Håkan Sandberg, Åke Lennander, Kersti Malmsten* and *all colleagues* at Mälardalens University who have encouraged and supported me throughout my studies although I mostly been conspicuous by my absence,
- *Marianne Carlsson, Per Lindberg, Harry Khamis and Bo Larsson* for valuable doctoral courses,
- *Ann-Britt Ivarsson* who always was there when I needed you the most,
- *Marie-Louise Schult, Margot Frisk, Birgitta Nätterlund, Helena Lindstedt* and *Anita Tollén*, my fellow doctoral students and occupational therapists, for inspiring discussions and support,
- *Kari Haave*, my best friend, for support and most important of all - giving me other things to do and think about,
- all friends in the "dog-world", giving me so much enjoy and perspective to the scientific world,
- my family, *Kristiina, John, Jörgen, Nils-Arne, Anneka, Kerstin, Anne, Ninni & Tomas, Pelle & Cilla* with families for being there with enjoyable, relaxing fellowship,
- *John* and *Jörgen* for helping me with the cover to the thesis,

and finally

- *Paul and Kajsa*, my husband and daughter, for your unfailing trust in me!

Financial support was given by the Vårdal Foundation, Mälardalens University and the Claes Groshinsky foundation.

REFERENCES

Adolfsson, Å., Råstam, L. (1992). Långtidssjukskrivna i Rosengård. En uppföljning efter fyra år. (Long-term sick-leave in Rosengård. A follow-up after four year). Försäkringskassan. (in Swedish)

Ahlgren, A., Hammarström, A. (2000). Back to work? Gendered experiences of rehabilitation. *Scandinavian Journal of Public Health*, **28**: 88-94.

Ahlström, G. (1994). *Consequences of Muscular Dystrophy: Impairment, Disability, Coping and Quality of Life*. Dissertation. University of Uppsala, Uppsala.

Aja, D. (1991). Occupational therapy intervention for overuse syndrome. *The American Journal of Occupational Therapy*, **45**:746-750.

Alexander, RW., Bradley, LA., Alarcon, GS., Triana-Alexander, M., Alberts, KR., Martin, MY., Stewart, KE. (1998). Sexual and physical abuse in women with fibromyalgia: association with outpatient health care utilization and pain medication. *Arthritis Care Research*, **11**: 102-115.

Alsop, A. Evidence-based practice and continuing professional development. *British Journal of Occupational Therapy*, **60**: 503-508.

Andersen, S., Worm-Pedersen, J. (1987). The prevalence of persistent pain in a Danish Population. *Pain*, suppl **4**:S322.

Andersson, C. (1997). Vem får rehabilitering? (Who gets rehabilitation?). *Miljön på jobbet*, **4**:19-23. (in Swedish)

Andersson, I., Ejlertsson, G., Leden, I., Rosenberg, C. (1993). Long-term pain in a geographically defined general population: Studies of differences in age, gender, social class, and pain localization. *Clinical Journal of Pain*, **9**:174-182.

Andersson, HI., Ejlertsson, G., Leden, I., Schersten, B. (1999a). Impact of chronic pain on health care seeking, self care, and medication. Results from a population-based Swedish study. *Journal of Epidemiological Community Health*, **53**: 503-509.

Andersson, HI., Ejlertsson, G., Leden, I., Schersten, B. (1999b). Musculoskeletal chronic pain in general practice. Studies of health care utilisation in comparison with pain prevalence. *Scandinavian Journal of Primary Health Care*, **17**: 87-92.

Arnstein, P., Caudill, M., Mandle, CL., Norris, A., Beasley, R. (1999). Self efficacy as a mediator of the relationship between pain intensity, disability and depression in chronic pain patients. *Pain*, **80**: 483-491.

Averill, PM., Novy, DM., Nelson, DV., Berry, LA. (1996). Correlates of depression in chronic pain patients: a comprehensive examination. *Pain*, **65**: 93-100.

Balacki, MF. (1988). Assessing mental health needs in the rural community: a critique of assessment approaches. *Issues of Mental Health Nursing*, **9**: 299-315.

Bellner, A-L. (1997). Professionalization and rehabilitation – the case of Swedish occupational och physical therapists. Linköping Studies in Arts and Science No. 166. Linköping University, Linköping.

Benn, SI., Peters, RS. (1964). *Principles of Political Thought*. New York: Colliers Books.

Björklund, A. (2000). On the Structure and Contents of Occupational Therapists Paradigms. Dissertation. Karolinska Institute, Stockholm. (in Swedish).

Blakeney, AB. (1984). Occupational therapy intervention in chronic pain. *Occupational Therapy in Health Care*, **1**:43-54.

Blyth, FM., March, LM., Brnabic, AJ., Jorm, LR., Williamson, M., Cousins, MJ. (2001). Chronic pain in Australia: a prevalence study. *Pain*, **89**: 127-134.

Bonica, JJ. (1953). The management of pain. Philadelphia: Lea & Febiger.

Brattberg, G., Thorslund, M., Wikman, A. (1988). 40 procent av Gävleborgs befolkning har långvariga smärtor. (40 percent of the inhabitants of Gävleborg have long-term pain) *Läkartidningen*, **85**: 4090-93. (in Swedish)

Brattberg, G., Thorslund, M., Wikman, A. (1989). The prevalence of pain in a general population, the results of a Postal survey in a county in Sweden. *Pain*, **37**: 215-222.

Brink, PM., Wood, MJ. (1989). *Advanced Design in Nursing Research*. Newbury Park: Sage Publication.

Bruhn, JG., Trevino, FM. (1979). A method for determining patients' perceptions of their health needs. *The Journal of Family Practice*, **8**: 809-818.

Bunston, T., Mackie, A., Jones, D., Mings, D. (1994). Identifying the nonmedical concerns of patients with ocular melanoma. *Journal of Ophthalmic Nursing & Technology*, **13**: No 5.

Bunston, T., Mings, D. (1995). Identifying the psychosocial needs of individuals with cancer. *Canadian Journal of Nursing Research*, **2**: 59-79.

Burnett, SE., Yerxa, EJ. (1980). Community based and college based needs assessment of physically disabled persons. *The American Journal of Occupational Therapy*, **34**: 201-207.

Carruthers, C. (1997). Developing a pain management programme. *British Journal of Occupational Therapy*, **60**: 221-222

Caruso, L.A., Chan, D.E. (1986). Evaluation and management of the patient with acute back pain. *American Journal of Occupational Therapy*. **40**: 347-351.

Christensen, C., Baum, C. (1997). *Occupational Therapy: Enabling, Function and Well-Being*. Thorofare, NJ: Slack, pp. 27-45, 590-528.

Chrubasik, S., Junck, H., Zappe, HA., Stutzke, O. (1998). A survey on pain complaints and health care utilization in a German population sample. *European Journal of Anaestesilogy*, **15**: 397-408.

Clark, F., Wood, W., Larson, EA. (1998). Occupational science: Occupational therapy's legacy for the 21st century. In: Neistadt, ME., Blesedell Crepeau, E. (eds.). *Occupational Therapy*. Philadelphia: Lippincott-Raven Publishers.

Crook, J., Rideout, E., Browne, G. (1984). The prevalence of pain complaints in a general population. *Pain*, **18**: 299-314.

Darnell, JL., Heater, SL. (1994). Occupational therapist or activity therapist – which do you choose to be? *The American Journal of Occupational Therapy*, **48**: 467-468.

Dragone, MA. (1990). Perspectives of chronically ill adolescents and parents on health care needs. *Pediatric Nursing*, **16**: 45-50, 108.

Engel, CC., von Korff, M., Katon, WJ. (1996). Back pain in primary care: predictors of high health-care costs. *Pain*, **65**: 197-204.

Erlandsson, LK., Eklund, M. (2001). Describing patterns of daily occupations – a methodological study comparing data from four different methods. *Scandinavian Journal of Occupational therapy*, **8**: 31-39.

Fast, C. (1995). Repetitive strain injury: An overview of the condition and its implications for occupational therapy practice. *Canadian Journal of Occupational Therapy*, **62**: 119-126.

Fishbain, DA., Rosomoff, H., Abdel-Moty, E., Saltzman, A., Steele-Rosomoff, R. (1996). "Movement" in Work Status After Pain Facility Treatment. *Spine*, **22**: 2662-2669.

Fishman Borelli, E., Warfield, CA. (1986). Occupational Therapy for Chronic Pain. *Hospital Practice*, **15**: 36K-37.

Flower, A., Naxon, E., Jones RE. (1981). An occupational therapy program for chronic back pain. *American Journal Occupational Therapy*. **35:** 243-248.

FSA (Förbundet Sveriges Arbetsterapeuter). (1983). Studiematerial för arbetsterapeuter. (Study material for occupational therapists, in Swedish). Nacka: Förbundet Sveriges Arbetsterapeuter.

Gaston-Johansson, F. (1985). Pain assessment with particular reference to pain terms, Instrument development and pain description. Dissertation. University of Göteborg, Göteborg.

Giacomini, MK., Cook, DJ., Satreiner, DL., Anand, SS. (2001). Guidelines as rationing tools: a qualitative analysis of psychosocial patient selection criteria for cardiac procedures. *CMAJ*, **164**: 634-640.

Gibson, L., Strong J. (1998). Assessment of psychosocial factors in functional capacity evaluation of clients with chronic back pain. *British Journal of Occupational Therapy*, **9**: 399-404.

Giles, GM., Allen, ME. (1986). Occupational therapy in the treatment of the patient with chronic pain. *British Journal of Occupational Therapy*, **49**: 4-9.

Heck, S. (1988). The effect of purposeful activity on pain tolerance. *The American Journal of Occupational Therapy*, **42**: 577 – 581.

Henriksson, C. (1995). *Living with fibromyalgia. A study of the consequences for daily activities*. Dissertation. Linköping University, Linköping.

Herbert, P., Rochman, DL. (1998). Treating the physical, psychological, and emotional aspects of patients with chronic pain. Dealing with pain. *Rehab Management*, **11**: 56, 58-59, 96.

Hinojosa, J., Kramer, P. (1997). Statement – fundamental concepts of occupational therapy: occupation, purposeful activity, and function. *The American Journal of Occupational Therapy*, **51**: 864-866.

Hopkins, HL., Smith, HD. (1993). *Willard and Spackman's Occupational Therapy. 8th ed.* Philadelphia: JB Lippincott Company. pp. 192-267, 596-603.

Houlding, AD., Wasserbauer, N. (1996). Psychosocial needs of older cancer patients: a pilot study abstract. *Medsurg Nursing*, **5**: 253-256.

Jacobs, K. (1999). Quick Reference Dictionary for Occupational Therapy (2nd edn.). Thorafare, NJ: Slack.

Jensen, I., Nygren, Å., Gamberale, F., Goldie, I., Westerholm, P. (1994) Coping with long-term musculoskeletal pain and its consequences: is gender a factor? *Pain*, **57**: 167-172.

Jensen, IB., Bodin, L., Ljungqvist., Bergström, GK., Nygren, Å. (2000) Assessing the needs of patients in pain: A matter of opinion? *Spine*, **25**: 2816-2823.

Jette, A.M., Davies, AR., Leary, PD., Calkings, DR., Rubenstein, LV., Fink, A., Kosecoff, J., Young, RT., Brook, RH., Delbanco, TL. (1986). The functional status questionnaire: reliability and validity when used in primary Care. *General Internal Medicine*, **1**: 143-149.

Joe, B.E. (1991). *Quality assurance on occupational therapy. A practioner's guide for setting up a QA system using three models*. USA: The American Occupational Therapy Association.

Johansson, EE., Hamberg, K., Westman, G., Lindgren G. (1999). The meanings of pain: an exploration of women's descriptions of symptoms. *Social Science & Medicine*, **48**: 1791-1802.

Johnson, JA. (1984). Occupational therapy and the patient with pain. *Occupational Therapy Health Care*. **1**: 7-15.Karasek, J R. (1979). Job demands, job decision latitude and mental strain: Implication for job redesign. *Administration Science Quarterly*, **24**: 285-307.

Karasek, JR. (1979). Job demands, job decision latitude and mental strain: Implication for job redesign. *Administration Science Quarterly*, **24**: 285-307.

Karasek, JR., Brisson, C., Kawakami, N., Houtman, I., Bongers, P., Amick, B. (1998). The Job Content Questionnaire (JCQ): An instrument for internationally comparative assessments of psychosocial job characteristics. *Journal of Occupational Health Psychology*, **3**: 322-355.

Karasek, JR., Theorell, T. (1990). *Healthy work: stress, productivity and the reconstruction of working life*. New York: Basic Books.

Karjalainen, K., Malmivaara, A., van Tulder, M., Ronie, R., Jauhianinen, M., Hurri, H., Koes, B. (2000). Multidisciplinary rehabilitation for fibromyalgia and musculoskeletal pain in working age adults (Cochrane Review). In: The Cochrane Library, Issue 1. Oxford: Update Software.

Kazdin, AE. (1998). *Research design in clinical psychology*. 3rd ed. Boston: Allyn and Bacon.

Kent, RM., Chandler, BJ., Barnes MP. (2000). An epidemiological survey of the health needs of disabled people in a rural community. *Clinical Rehabilitation*, **14**: 481-490.

Kielhofner, G. (1992). *Conceptual foundations of occupational therapy*. Philadelphia: F.A. Davis Company.

Kiernan, M., Winkleby, MA. (2000). Identifying patients for weight-loss treatment: an empirical evaluation of the NHLBI obesity education initiative expert panel recommendations. *Archive Internal Medicine*, **160**: 2169-2176.

Klayman-Callahan, D. (1993). Work hardening for a client with low back pain. *The American Journal of Occupational Therapy*, **47**: 645-649.

Kresten, P., George, S., McLellan, L., Smith, JA., Mullee, MA. (2000). Disabled people and professionals differ in their perception of rehabilitation needs. *Journal of Public Health Medicine*, **22**: 393-399.

Lawton, L. (1999). Approaches to Needs Assessment. In: Perkins, ER., Simnett, I., Wright, L. (eds). *Evidence-based health promotion*. John Wiley & Sons Ltd.

Lazarus, RS. (1991). *Emotion and adaptation*. New York: Oxford University Press.

Lazarus, R.S., Folkman, S. (1984). *Stress, Appraisal and Coping*. New York: Springer.

Lindström, I-L. (1990). *Utveckling av arbetsterapeutyrket under de senaste 50 åren*. (The development of the occupational therapist' profession during the latest 50 years.) Arbetsterapeuten publicerar sig nr 1. Stockholm: Förbundet Sveriges Arbetsterapeuter. (in Swedish)

Linton, SJ. (2000). A review of psychological risk factors in back and neck pain. *Spine*, **25**: 1148-1156.

Linton, SJ., Hallden, K. (1998). Can we screen for problematic back pain? A screening questionnaire for predicting outcome in acute and subacute back pain. *Clinical Journal of Pain*, **14**: 209-215.

Linton, SJ., Hellsing, AL., Hallden, K. (1998). A population-based study of spinal pain among 35-45-year-old individuals. Prevalence, sick leave, and health care use. *Spine*, **23**: 1457-1463.

Linton, SJ., Ryberg, M. (2000). Do epidemiological results replicate? The prevalence and health-economic consequences of neck and back pain in the general population. *European Journal of Pain*, **4**: 347-54.

Liss, PE. (1990). Health Care Need - Meaning and Measurements. Dissertation. Linköping University, Linköping.

Lund, A., Andersson-Nordberg, B. (1998*). Arbetsterapins perspektiv och innehåll i Sverige under åren 1970 – 1993*. (The perspective and content in occupational therapy in Sweden during 1970-1993). Arbetsterapeuten publicerar sig nr 5. Stockholm: Förbundet Sveriges Arbetsterapeuter.

Löfgren, B. (1999). Rehabilitation of old people with stroke. Outcome prediction and long-term follow-up. Dissertation. Umeå University, Umeå.

Manderbacka, K. (1998). Questions on survey questions on health. Dissertation. Stockholm University, Stockholm.

Matthew, G.K. (1971). Measuring need and evaluating services. In *Problems and progress in medical care,* 6th Series McLaclan, G. Ed. pp. 27-46. U.S. Portfolio for Health. New York: Oxford University Press.

McCormack, G. (1988). Pain management by occupational therapists. *The American Journal of Occupational Therapy,* **42**: 582–590.

McLaughlin Gray, J. (2001). Discussion of the ICIDH-2 in relation to occupational therapy and occupational science. *Scandinavian Journal of Occupational Therapy,* **8**: 1-30.

Medline. Draft. (web page) http://www4.mcbo.nlm.nih.gov/htbin-post/Entrez/meshbrowser. (accessed 19 November). 2000.

Merskey, H. (ed) International Association for the study of Pain. (1979). Pain terms: a list with definitions and notes on usage. *Pain,* **6**: 249-252.

Merskey, H. (1996). Pain specialists and pain terms. *Pain,* **64**: 205.

Mosey, AC. (1974). An alternative: the biopsychosocial model. *American Journal of Occupational Therapy,* **28**: 137-140.

Mosey, AC. (1996). *Psychosocial components of occupational therapy.* Philadelphia: Lippincott-Raven Publishers.

Müllersdorf, M., Söderback, I. (1998). Needs assessment methods in healthcare and rehabilitation. *Critical Reviews in Physical and Rehabilitation Medicine,* **10**: 57-73.

Nelson, DL. (1997). Why the profession of occupational therapy will flourish in the 21st century. *The American Journal of Occupational Therapy,* **51**: 11-24.

Nordenskiöld, U. (1996). Daily activities in women with rheumatoid arthritis. Dissertation. Göteborg University, Göteborg.

Novy, DM., Nelson, DV., Averill, PM., Berry, LA. (1996). Gender differences in the expression of depressive symptoms among chronic pain patients. *Clinical Journal of Pain,* **12**: 23-29.

Nätterlund, B. (2001) Living with muscular dystrophy. Dissertation. Uppsala University, Uppsala.

Nätterlund, B., Ahlström G. (1999). Problem-focused coping and satisfaction in individuals with muscular dystrophy and post-polio. *Scandinavian Journal of Caring Science,* **13**: 26-32.

O'Hara, M. (1992). Occupational therapy and the pain management team. *British Journal of Occupational Therapy.* **55**: 19-20.

Percy-Smith, J. (1996). *Needs assessments in public policy.* Buckingham, U.K.: Open University Press.

Persson, D., Erlandsson, L-K., Eklund, M., Iwarsson, S. (2001). Value dimensions, meaning, and complexity in human occupation – a tentative structure for analysis. *Scandinavian Journal of Occupational therapy,* **8**: 7-18.

Philips, ME., Bruehl, S., Harden, RN. (1997). Work-related post-traumatic stress disorder: Use of exposure therapy in work-simulation activities. *The American Journal of Occupational Therapy,* **51**: 696-700.

Polit, D., Hungler, B. *Nursing research - Principles and Methods.* (1995). 5th ed. Philadelphia: Lippingcott Company.

Rebeiro, KL. (1998). Occupation – as means to mental health: A review of the literature, and a call for research. *Canadian Journal of Occupational Therapy,* **65**: 12-19.

Reed, KL., Sanderson, SN. (1999). Concepts of occupational therapy (4th ed). Philadelphia; Lippincott Williams & Wilkins. pp 51-62; 342-373.

Reviere, R., Carter, C., Neuschats, S. (1994). Longitudinal needs assessment: Aging in a suburban community. *Physical & Occupational Therapy in Geriatrics,* **12**: 1-15.

Riegelman, K., Hirsch, R. (1996). *Studying a study and testing a test.* 3rd ed. London: Little Brown & Company.

Royce, D., Drude, K. (1982). Mental health needs assessment: beware of false promises. Community Mental Health Journal, **18**: 97-106.

Rubenstein, LV., Calkins, DR., Young, RT., Cleary, PD., Fink, A., Kosecoff, J., Jette, AM., Davies, AR., Delbanco, TL., Brook, RH. (1989). Improving patient function: a randomized trial of functional disability screening. *Annual Internal Medicine,* **111**: 836-842.

Rustia, J., Hartley, R., Hansen, G., Schulte, D., and Spielman, L. (1984). Redefinition of school nursing practice: integrating the developmentally disabled. *Journal of School Health,* 58-62.

SBU. (1991). Swedish Council on Technology Assessment in Health Care. Ont I ryggen – orsaker, diagnostik och behandling (Back pain – causes, diagnosis and treatment). Stockholm: Statens Beredning för medicinsk Utvärdering. (in Swedish).

SBU. (2000). Swedish Council on Technology Assessment in Health Care. Ont i ryggen, ont i nacken. Volym I, II. (Back Pain, Neck Pain. An evidence Based Review) Stockholm: SB Offset AB, 2000. (in Swedish)

Schut, HA., Stam HJ. (1994). Goals in rehabilitation teamwork. *Disability and Rehabilitation,* **16**: 223-226.

Scudds, RA., Solomon, P. (1995). Pain curriculum for students in occupational therapy or physical therapy. *Physiotherapy Canada,* **2**: 79-84.

Simeone, R., Frank, B., Aryan, Z. (1993). Needs assessment in substance misuse: a comparison of approaches and case study. *International Journal of Addiction,* **28**: 767-792.

Skov, T., Borg, V., Orhede, E. (1996). Psychosocial and physical risk factors for musculoskeletal disorders of the neck, shoulders, and lower back in salespeople. *Occupational Environment Medicine,* **53**: 351-6.

Spertus, IL., Burns, J., Glenn, B., Lofland, K., McCracken, L. (1999). Gender differences in associations between trauma history and adjustment among chronic pain patients. *Pain,* **82**: 97-102.

Soriano F. (1995). *Conducting needs assessments - a multidisciplinary approach.* Thousand Oaks: Sage Publications.

SOS. (1997). The Swedish National Board of Health and Welfare. Behandling av långvarig smärta, (Treatment of long-term pain). (SOS 1994:4). Stockholm: Socialstyrelsen. (in Swedish)

SOS. (1999). The Swedish National Board of Health and Welfare. Prioriteringar i sjukvården. Beslut och tillämpning. *(Priorities in health care. Decisions and applications.)* (SOS 1999:16). Stockholm: Socialstyrelsen. (in Swedish)

SOU. (1995). Prioriteringsutredningens slutbetänkande. Vårdens svåra val. (The difficult choices in health care). (SOU 1995:5). Stockholm: Socialdepartementet. (in Swedish)

SOU. (2000). The Swedish Ministry of Health and Social Affairs (2000). Slutbetänkande av utredningen om Den arbetslivsinriktade rehabiliteringen (Rehabilitation to work). (SOU 2000:78). Stockholm: Socialdepartementet (in Swedish).

Statistical Package for Social Science (SPSS). (1998). SPSS Base, advanced statistics, professional statistics 8.0 for Windows, SPSS Scandinavia AB, Stockholm, Chicago, Illinois, USA

Statistical Package for Social Science (SPSS). (1999). SPSS base, advanced statistics, professional statistics 9.0 for Windows, SPSS Scandinavia AB, Stockholm, Chicago, Illinois, USA.

Stein, F., Roose, B. (2000). Pocket guide to treatment in occupational therapy. San Diego: Singular Publishing Group Thomson Learning.

Sternbach, RA. (1986) Survey of pain in the United States: the Nuprin Pain Report. *Clinical Journal of Pain,* **1**:49-53.

Strong, J. (1986). Occupational therapy's contribution to pain management in Queensland. *Australian Occupational Therapy Journal,* **33**: 101-107.

Strong, J. (1987). Chronic pain management: the occupational therapist's role. *British Journal of Occupational Therapy,* **50**: 262-263.

Strong, J. (1989). The occupational therapist's contribution to the management of chronic pain. *Patient Management,* **13**: 43-50.

Strong, J. (1991). Relaxation training and chronic pain. *British Journal of Occupational Therapy,* **54**: 216-218.

Strong, J. (1996). *Chronic pain. The occupational therapists perspective.* New York: Churchill Livingstone.

Strong, J. (1998). Incorporating cognitive-behavioural therapy with occupational therapy: A comparative study with patients with low back pain. *Journal of Occupational Rehabilitation,* **1**: 61-71

Strong, J., Ashton, R. and Large, RG. (1994). Function and the patient with chronic low back pain. *Clinical Journal of Pain,* **10**: 191-96.

Szpalski, M., Nordin, M., Skovron, ML., Melot, C., Cukier, D. (1995). Health care utilization for low back pain in Belgium. Influence of sociocultural factors and health beliefs. *Spine,* **20**: 431-442.

Söderback, I. (1993) *Kvalitetssäkring inom arbetsterapi* (Quality insurance within occupational therapy), Stockholm: Spri.

Söderback, I., Hammersly Paulsson, E. (1997). Nurses judgement of the need for occupational therapy in acute cancer care. *Cancer Nursing,* **19**: 267 - 73.

Söderback, I., Pettersson, I., von Essen, L., Stein, F. (2000). Cancer patients' and their physicians' perceptions of the formers' need for occupational therapy. *Scandinavian Journal of Occupational Therapy,* **7**: 77-86.

Söderback, I., Schult, M-L., Nordemar, R. (1993). Assessment of patients with chronic back pain using the "Functional Status Questionnaire". *Scandinavian Journal of Rehabilitation Medicine,* **25**: 139-143.

Tabachnick, BG., Fidell, LS. (1996). *Using Multivariate Statistics.* 3rd ed. New York: Harper Collins Publishers Inc.

The American Psychiatric Association. (1994). *Diagnostic and statistic manual of mental disorders. 4th ed.* American psychiatric press, Inc.

The Swedish National Board of Health and Welfare. (1997). Swedish version of the International Classification of Diseases, 10th Revision. Klassifikation av sjukdomar och hälsoproblem 1997, Primärvård. Socialstyrelsen. Stockholm: Nordstedts Tryckeri. (in Swedish

The National Swedish Social Insurance Board. (1999). Equality when facing the social insurance office? Lika inför kassan? Riksförsäkringsverket. Stockholm. (in Swedish).

Theorell, T., Harms-Ringdahl, K., Ahlberg-Hultén, G., Westin, B. (1991). Psychosocial job factors and symptoms from the locomotor system - a multicausal analysis. *Scandinavian Journal of Rehabilitation Medicine,* **23**: 165-173.

Theorell, T., Nordemar, R., Michélsen, H., Stockholm Music I Study Group. (1993). Pain thresholds during standardized psychological stress in relation to perceived psychosocial work situation. *Journal of Psychosomatic Research,* **37**: 299-305.

Tjornov, J. (1987). *Ergoterapi. Baggrund og udvikling.* Kopenhavn: Foreningen af dansek laegestuderende forlag.

Tollén, A., Ahlström, G. (1998). Assessment instrument for problem-focused coping. Reliability test of APC. Part 1. *Scandinavian Journal of Caring Sciences,* **12**: 18-24.

Trombly, C. (1995). Occupation: Purposefulness and meaningfulness as therapeutic mechanism. *The American Journal of Occupational Therapy,* **49**: 960-972.

Turk, DC., Okifuji, A. (1998). Treatment of chronic pain patients: clinical outcomes, cost-effectiveness, and cost-benefits of multidisciplinary pain centres. *Critical Reviews in Physical and Rehabilitation Medicine,* **2**: 81-202.

Turner, JA., LeResche, L., Von Korff, M., Ehrlich, K. (1998). Back pain in primary care. Patient characteristics, content of initial visit, and short-term outcomes. *Spine,* **23**: 463-469.

Törnquist, K. (1995). Att fastställa och mäta förmåga till dagliga livets aktiviteter (ADL). (Verifying and measuring the ability to perform activities of daily living [ADL]). Dissertation. Göteborg University, Göteborg. (in Swedish).

Zitman, FG., Linssen, AC., Van, HR. (1992). Chronic pain beyond patienthood. *Journal of Nerv Mental Disorders,* **180**: 97-100.

van Oel, CJ., Schmidt, SH., Oort-Marburger, D. (1995). The impact of job characteristics on work-related well-being of handicapped employees in relation to pain. *Clinical Rehabilitation,* **9**: 254-26.

Velozo, CA. (1993). Work evaluations: critique of the state of the art of functional assessment of work. *American Journal of Occupational Therapy,* **47**: 203-209.

Ventura, DL., Flinn-Wagner, S.R. (1997). Non-work issues that affect successful return to work for upper extremity injured employees. *Work.* **8**: 73-75.

Ward, MM. (1997). Rheumatology visit frequency and changes in functional disability and pain in patients with rheumatoid arthritis. *The Journal of Rheumatology,* **24**: 35-42.

Warms, CA. (1987). Health promotion services in post-rehabilitation spinal cord injury health care. *Rehabilitation Nursing,* **12**: 304-308.

Weir, R., Browne, G., Tunks, E., Gafni, A., Roberts, J. (1996). Gender differences in psychosocial adjustment to chronic pain and expenditures for health care services used. *The Clinical Journal of Pain,* **12**: 277-290.

Wilkin, D. (1993).The measurement of needs and outcomes: aids to enhancing shared understanding between doctors and patients. *Scandinavian Journal of Primary Health Care,* **11**: Suppl 1: 36-39.

Wiskin, LF. (1998). Cognitive-behavioural therapy: a psychoeducational treatment approach for the American worker with rheumatoid arthritis. *Work,* **10**: 41-48.

WHO. (1998). The International Classification of Impairments, Disabilities, and Handicaps. Draft (web page) http://www.who.ch/whosis/icidh.htm (accessed 23 June 1998).

WHO. (2000). The International Classification to Functioning, Disability and Health. ICIDH-2. Prefinal Draft December 2000 (web page) http://www.who.int/icidh. (Accessed 23 March 2001).

Wright, CC., Whittington D. (1992) *Quality Assurance. An introduction for health care professionals.* New York: Churchill Livingstone.

Wright, J., Williams, R., Wilkinson, JR. (1998). Health needs assessment. Development and importance of health needs assessment. *BMJ,* **316**:1310-1313.

The items in the questionnaire "Pain and occupations" used in Study II-III

No	Item	Response options
	Demography	
1	Gender	1) man; 2) women
2	Age	1) years
3	Native country	1) Sweden; 2) other
4	Civil status	1) single; 2) married/cohabit; 3) widow/widower; 4) divorced
5	Education	1) < 7 years; 2) 7-9 years; 3) 10-12 years; 4) >13 years
6	Housing	1) owned house; 2) rented house; 3) flat – cooperative; 4) flat – with right of tenancy; 5) other arrangement
	Pain	
7	For how long do you have had pain?	1) 3-6 months; 2) more than 6 months
8	Do you have pain more or less all the time?	1) yes; 2) no
9	Is the pain regularly recurrent?	1) yes; 2) no
10	Is the pain temporarily?	1) yes; 2) no
11	Have you got any diagnose from a physician?	1) yes; 2) no
12	If yes, which diagnosis?	open answer
13	Which description would best describe your pain?	1) pain; 2) marked pain; 3) severe pain
14 – 23	*Where is the pain located?* 14) head, face, mouth; 15) neck; 16) shoulder, arms;.17) chest; 18) abdomen; 19) pelvis; 20) upper back; 21) lower back; 22) hips; 23) legs	1) yes; 2) no
24 - 32	*How would you describe the pain?* 24) burning; 25) searing; 26) sharp; 27) gnawing; 28) spasmodic; 29) aching; 30) sore; 31) tensed; 32) pricking	1) yes; 2) no
33 - 43	*Have you sometime felt due to pain?* 33) depressed; 34) worried; 35) anxious; 36) sensible; 37) irritated; 38) distressed; 39) easily tired; 40) lack of initiative; 41) loss of appetite; 42) isolated; 43) sensitive	1) never; 2) sometimes; 3) often; 4) all the time
44 - 51	*Have you sometime had due to pain?* 44) sleeplessness; 45) difficult to relax; 46) nightmares; 47) stress feelings; 48) irresolution; 49) inferiority feelings; 50) difficult to concentrate; 51) difficulty with memory	1) never; 2) sometimes; 3) often; 4) all the time
	Occupations in daily life *(Parts of the "Functional Status Questionnaire")*	
52	*Have you during the previous month been able to:* Take care of yourself, that is, eating or bathing?	1) without problems; 2) some problems: 3) big problems; 4) not performed due to health; 5) not performed due to other reasons
53	Stand up from/sit down on the chair or lay down on the bed?	as above
54	Take a quite long walk (several blocks)?	as above
55	Take a shorter walk (one block)?	as above

Continued: The items in the questionnaire "Pain and occupations" used in Study II-III

	Continued: **Occupations in daily life**	*Response options*
56	Walk up the stairs?	1) without problems; 2) some problems: 3) big problems; 4) not performed due to health; 5) not performed due to other reasons
57	Walk indoors e.g. in home?	as above
58	Perform housework (e.g. clean, repair)?	as above
59	Go for an errand e.g. shopping?	as above
60	Drive a car?	as above
61	Go by public means?	as above
62	Perform more demanding activity such as run, lift heavy things, heavier gardening or participate in some demanding sport?	as above
63	What is your opinion about your health status?	1) very satisfying; 2) satisfying; 3) unsatisfying; 4) very unsatisfying
64	Estimate the number of days that you have not performed paid work and/or other daily occupations you should or wanted to do?	1) number of days
	How much of your time during the previous month have you had difficulties to:	
65	Visit family and friends?	1) no time; 2) some time; 3) almost all the time; 4) all the time; 5) not done of other reasons
66	Participate in activities as social life or club activities?	as above
67	Take care of others, e.g. family?	as above
68	How often during the previous month did you meet friends and relatives, e.g. went out together, visited each other, talked on telephone?	1) every day; 2) a couple of days per week; 3) once a week; 4) 2-3 times per month; 5) once a month; 6) not at all
69	Which of the options describes best your actual work-situation during the previous month? (except housework)	1) working fulltime; 2) working part time; 3) Other situation such as…..
	How much of the time during the previous month:	
70	Did you work as much as other workmates with similar tasks?	1) never; 2) sometime; 3) almost all the time; 4) all the time
71	Did you work in short periods or did breaks due to your health?	as above
72	Did you work as much time as you use to do?	as above
73	Could you perform your work tasks with accuracy and precision as other workmates with similar tasks?	as above
74	Did you perform your ordinary work tasks but with some changes due to your health, e.g. with special equipment or ex-changing work tasks with other workmates?	as above
75	Have you been worried to loose your work due to your health?	as above
	Coping *(Parts of the "Assessment of Problem-focused Coping")*	
	Have you any special ways to perform tasks you want/ have to in spite of pain?	
76	Compensating by tricks or stratagems	1) never; 2) sometimes; 3) often; 4) always
77	Technical aids	as above
78	Own technical solutions	as above
79	Leaving the task or getting help from others	as above
80	Avoiding the task	as above
81	Perform the task partly	as above

Continues: The items in the questionnaire "Pain and occupations" used in Study II-III

Work *(Parts of the "Swedish modified version of the demand/control questionnaire")*		*Response options*
82	It's a calm and pleasant atmosphere on my workplace	1) definitely true; 2) partly true; 3) mostly not true; 4) not at all true
83	It's a good cohesion	as above
84	My workmates are supporting me	as above
85	My workmates are understanding if I have a bad day	as above
86	I am at ease with my workmates	as above
87	Does your work tasks demand a very rapid tempo?	as above
88	Does your work tasks demand very heavy work?	as above
89	Does your work tasks demand a great effort?	as above
90	Do you have enough of time to be able to perform the work tasks?	as above
91	Are there contradictory demands at your work?	as above
92	Do you learn new things at work?	as above
93	Do you have to be skilful at work?	as above
94	Do you have to be innovative at work?	as above
95	Do you perform the same work tasks over and over again?	as above
96	Have you possibility to decide how your work tasks will be performed?	as above
97	Have you possibility to decide what work task that will be performed at your work?	as above

Treatments

What treatments have you been recommended by health care (physicians or other health care staff) or have arranged on own initiative?

| 98 – 128 | 98) surgical operation; 99) medicines; 100) rest /confined to bed; 101) corset, orthoses, bandage; 102) stretching muscular; 103) thermo-treatment; 104) cryotherapy ; 105) manipulation of joints; 106) massage; 107) electrical treatment; 108) acupuncture; 109) physical activation at home; 110) physical activation in training halls; 111) relaxation training; 112) body awareness training; 113) bio-feed-back; 114) ergonomic counselling; 115) ergonomic practical education; 116) education about pain; 117) change of the work – environment; 118) change of work – organisation; 119) social welfare officer, family-therapy; 120) psychological support; 121) special psycho-therapy; 122) zone therapy; 123) music therapy; 124) meditation/yoga; 125) Feldenkreis/Rosen therapy; 126) nature cure medicine; 127) clergyman/priest or other church contact, confession; 128) New Age alternative | Been recommended: 1) never; 2) entered and fulfilled; 3) not entered or not fulfilled. Arranged on own initiative: 1) fulfilled; 2) not fulfilled |

Health care institutions

What health care-institutions have you visited due to pain?

| 128-133 | 128) primary care; 129) county hospital; 130) regional hospital; 131) rehabilitation clinic; 132) pain clinic; 133) private clinic | 1) yes; 2) no |

Health care staff

From whom have you got treatment for your pain?

| 134-142 | 134) physician; 135) nurse; 136) occupational therapist; 137) welfare officer; 138) psychologist; 139) physiotherapist; 140) chiropractor; 141) vocational guidance officer; 142) clergyman, priest | 1) yes; 2) no |

Results of principal component analyses of "emotional/affective effects of pain" -items in the questionnaire "Pain and occupations" used in Study II-III

Item		Study II			Study III		
		Factor number	Factor loading	% explained variance	Factor number	Factor loading	% explained variance
Pain (emotional/affective effects of pain)							
Insufficiency	Inferiority feelings	1[1]	0.75	42.0	1[3]	0.75	31.1
	Irresolution	1	0.73		1	0.75	
	Difficulty with memory	1	0.72		1	0.72	
	Nightmares	1	0.68		1	0.66	
	Stress feelings	1	0.52		2[4]	0.50	24.5
Restlessness[2]	Diff to relax	2[2]	0.80	14.5	2	0.79	
	Sleeplessness	2	0.77		2	0.76	
	Diff to concentrate	2	0.66		2	0.61	

[1-4]Cronbach Alpha Coefficients: [1](0.77); [2](0.66): [3](0.74); [4](0.69)

Item		Study II			Study III		
		Factor number	Factor loading	% explained variance	Factor number	Factor loading	% explained variance
Pain (emotional/affective effects of pain)							
Dispirited	Loss of appetite	1[1]	0.77	42.4	1[4]	0.77	22.3
	Isolated	1	0.73		1	0.75	
	Sensitive	1	0.64		1	0.66	
	Lack of initiative	1	0.62		1	0.60	
Anxious	Worried	2[2]	0.82	10.1	2[5]	0.80	20.9
	Anxious	2	0.78		2	0.76	
	Distressed	2	0.72		2	0.71	
Depressed	Irritated	3[3]	0.81	9.3	3[6]	0.80	17.3
	Easily tired	3	0.62		3	0.64	
	Depressed	3	0.62		3	0.59	
	Sensible	3	0.49		1	0.43	

[1-4]Cronbach Alpha Coefficients: [1](0.74); [2](0.78): [3](0.72); [4](0.78); [5](0.75); [6](0.61)

Item	Study II			Study III		
	Factor number	Factor loading	% explained variance	Factor number	Factor loading	% explained variance
Coping						
Avoids the task	1[1]	0.83	29.4	1[3]	0.84	27.8
Performs the task partly	1	0.83		1	0.81	
Leaving the task/getting help from others	1	0.48		1	0.52	
Own technical solution	2[2]	0.71	16.6	2[4]	0.74	
Compensating by tricks or stratagems	2	0.54		2	0.56	19.0
Technical aids	2	0.48		2	0.48	

[1-4]Cronbach Alpha Coefficients: [1](0.75); [2](0.45): [3](0.76); [4](0.62)

Results of principal component analysis of the "treatment"-items in the questionnaire "Pain and occupations" used in Study II-III

Item	Study II			Study III		
	Factor number	Factor loading	% explained variance	Factor number	Factor loading	% explained variance
Physical treatments/training (0.82) [1]				**(0.82)** [1]		
Electrical treatment	1	0.72	11.65	1	0.71	11.90
Massage	1	0.72		1	0.73	
Thermo-treatment	1	0.69		1	0.70	
Stretching muscular	1	0.64		1	0.65	
Acupuncture	1	0.61		1	0.62	
Manipulation of joints (by chiropractor /naprapath)	1	0.58		1	0.59	
Physical activation at home	1	0.55		1	0.54	
Physical activation in training halls	1	0.50		1	0.47	
Alternative treatments (0.62) [1]				**(0.68)** [1]		
New-Age-alternative [3]	2	0.72	7.00	2	0.72	8.20
Music therapy [3]	2	0.71		2	0.69	
Clergyman/priest or other church contact, confession [3]	2	0.51		2	0.62	
Zone therapy [3]	2	0.43		2	0.53	
Feldenkreis/Rosen therapy [3]	2	0.35		2	0.40	
Ergonomics (0.65) [1]				**(0.65)** [1]		
Ergonomic counselling	3	0.69	6.77	3	0.69	6.68
Change of the work - environment	3	0.67		3	0.69	
Ergonomic practical education	3	0.66		3	0.66	
Change of work organisation	3	0.57		3	0.59	
Psychological support (0.61) [1]				**(0.62)** [1]		
Psychological support	4	0.75	6.13	4	0.74	5.96
Social welfare officer, family-therapy	4	0.66		4	0.66	
Special psychotherapy	4	0.57		4	0.57	
Medical treatment (0.53) [1]				**(0.47)** [1]		
Surgical operation	5	0.71	5.63	6	0.76	5.30
Medicines	5	0.59		6	0.33	
Rest/confined to bed	5	0.55		6	0.35	
Corset, orthoses, bandage	5	0.53		6	0.61	
Other [2]						
Body awareness training	6	0.71	5.16	5	0.74	5.30
Relaxation training	6	0.56		5	0.54	
Bio-feed-back	7	0.63	4.54			
Meditation/Yoga	7	0.53		2	0.53	
Nature cure medicine	8	0.68	4.07	7	0.74	4.33
Cold-treatment	8	0.34		7	0.35	

[1] Cronbach's Alpha Coefficients; [2] No tests for internal consistency performed

The items and results of Principal Component Analysis in the questionnaire "Occupational Therapy Needs Assessment – Pain" (OTNA-P) used in Study IV

No	Item	Factor number	Factor loading	% explained variance
1	Do you consider that the patient have decreased ability to perform the daily occupations that she/he wish or have to due to pain?	-	-	-
1b	If yes, is it caused by pain in: 1.1) head, face, mouth; 1.2) neck; 1.3) shoulder, arms; 1.4) chest; 1.5) abdomen; 1.6) pelvis; 1.7) upper back; 1.8) lower back; 1.9) hips; 1.10) legs			
2	What activity-limitation would you consider be the main problem for the patient ?	-	-	-
Need for education (0.71) [1]				
6	Has the patient difficulties to <u>adjust to</u> the physical and/or psychological changes which occur due to pain?	1	0.82	15.64
5	Has the patient need of <u>more knowledge</u> about pain?	1	0.73	
8	Is the patient <u>more tensed and/or suffering from stress</u> when she/he has pain?	1	0.72	
9	Has the patient any need of <u>learning new ways</u> to e.g. lift and carry things to be able to perform his/hers work tasks in a better way despite pain?	1	0.64	
Needs due to limitations in activity performance (0.63) [1]				
14	Does it happen that the patient due to pain has to <u>interrupt</u> the performance of activities (e.g. work, hobbies, housework)?	2	0.82	15.38
13	Does the patient get <u>more pain</u> at work or when performing housework?	2	0.74	
16	Is it with <u>more effort</u> that the patient performs daily occupations compared to when he/she did not have pain?	2	0.67	
15	Has the patient due to pain <u>give up</u> activities that he/she would like to do (e.g. work, hobbies, housework)?	2	0.58	
18	Do you assess that the pain restrains the patient to live up to the existing <u>expectations</u> on him/her at work (e.g. as work-mate, work manager) or in private (e.g. as parent, husband/wife)?	2	0.46	
Needs due to discouragement (0.66) [1]				
4	Has the patient any need <u>support/counselling to take up activities</u> again that she/he previously performed but gave up due to pain?	3	0.76	11.86
10	Has the patient been forced to <u>stop perform</u> activities that are valuable for him/her due to pain?	3	0.61	
12	Do you consider that the patients <u>self-confidence to his/her ability</u> to perform daily occupations has decreased due to pain?	3	0.59	
11	Do you assess that the patient disposal on personal care – housework – work – leisure – rest/sleep is <u>unbalanced</u> concerning time?	3	0.38	
Need as an effect of dependency				
7	Is the patient <u>dependent of others</u> to be able to perform daily occupations (e.g. to shop, to lift, to carry)?	4	0.77	10.51
Work related needs (0.40) [1]				
17	If the patient is on sick-leave: Do you assess it valuable for the patient <u>to be on his/hers workplace</u> and work without demands on work-performance, in order to maintain contact with the work and/or to decrease passiveness?	5	0.77	10.24
3	Has the patient any need of <u>adaptation or changes</u> made on her/his workplace/home to be able to perform work tasks in a better way (e.g. adaptation of table height, change chair)?	5	0.63	

- = not included in the factor analysis; [1] Cronbach Alpha Coefficients

The results of Principal Component Analysis of the questionnaire "Occupational Therapy Needs Assessment – Pain" (OTNA-P) used in Study V

No	Item	Factor number	Factor loading	% explained variance
Limitations in activity performance (0.89)[1]				28.30
14	Interrupt performance of activities due to pain	1	0.84	
15	Give up activities due to pain	1	0.84	
16	Perform activities with more effort	1	0.78	
7	Dependent of others	1	0.69	
10	Stopped performing activities	1	0.69	
12	Deficient self-confidence	1	0.64	
13	More pain in activity	1	0.61	
18	Difficulties with perceived expectations	1	0.57	
Need for education (0.57)[1]				11.86
5	Need of more knowledge about pain	2	0.70	
9	Need to learn new ways to handle activities	2	0.70	
17	Would like to be at workplace during sick-leave	2	0.54	
8	Tensed/stressed due to pain	2	0.40	
Need to regain activities (0.56)[1]				
3	Need of changes in home or at workplace	3	-0.74	10.49
4	Need of support to regain activities	3	-0.73	
Adjustment difficulties (0.50)[1]				
11	Temporal imbalance concerning rest/work/leisure	4	0.87	8.96
6	Difficulties to adjust to changes	4	0.35	

[1] Cronbach Alpha Coefficients

The list of suggested areas in occupational therapy attached to OTNA-P used in (Study IV)

No	Areas
1	Personal self-care
2	Housework
3	Work / school
4	Leisure
5	Psychosocial factors
6	Environmental factors

The list of suggested interventions in occupational therapy attached to OTNA-P and the results of the principal component analyses (used in Study IV)

No	Interventions	Factor number	Factor loading	% explained variance
Education and stress management (0.83) [1]				
10	Stress management	1	0.77	17.09
12	Pain education	1	0.72	
9	Relaxation techniques	1	0.71	
16	Attitudes about pain – modify	1	0.64	
15	Attitudes about pain – assessment	1	0.61	
21	Use of biofeedback, TNS	1	0.54	
2	Goal setting (interaction between the patient and therapist)	1	0.48	
Behavioral interventions (0.70) [1]				
13	Pain reporting/diary	2	0.43	11.20
1	Assessment task performance/activity analysis	2	0.71	
8	Ergonomics – training in daily occupations	2	0.69	
11	Energy conservation	2	0.62	
7	Body mechanics training	2	0.49	
5	Work conditioning and work hardening	2	0.44	
3	Counselling	2	0.42	
Hand-treatment (0.62) [1]				
20	Splinting	3	0.79	8.70
19	Joint protection – education	3	0.68	
Group activities (0.69) [1]				
4	Group activities/counselling	4	0.78	8.63
14	Back school – education of the function of the back	4	0.71	
Activity tolerance (0.59) [1]				
23	Use of arts and crafts	5	0.77	7.67
6	Activity tolerance/endurance	5	0.71	
22	Use of for the patient purposeful activities	5	0.52	
External adaptations (0.46) [1]				
18	Adaptation of environment	6	0.72	6.97
17	Assistive devices enabling/simplifying daily occupations	6	0.53	

[1] Cronbach Alpha Coefficients

Questionnaire concerning specific pain-related characteristics

Characteristics	*Response option*
Gender	man; women
Age	18-19; 20-29; 30-39; 40-49; 50-58 years
Education	< 7; 7-9; 10-12; >13 years
Had previous long-term/recurrent pain (> 3 months)?	yes; no
Had previous long sick-leave periods (> 3 months) due to pain?	yes; no

Please answer the questions on the circumstances you perceived during the previous month

Is your pain searing, aching or gnawing pain?	never; sometimes (1-2 / week); often (3-4 times/week); always (5-7 times/week)
Do you have pain in shoulders/lower back?	as above
Do you have difficulties to perform daily occupations due to pain?	as above

Have you due to pain:

been easily tired	as above
felt restlessness	as above
been depressed	as above
been irresolute	as above
Have you had repeated work task, e.g. do the same tasks over and over again?	as above
Do you need of changes at work place due to pain (e.g. change of work tasks or physical work environment)?	none; some; few; many; don't have a job